THE
COLLAGEN
GLOW

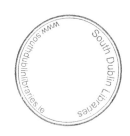

THE
COLLAGEN
GLOW

A GUIDE TO INGESTIBLE SKINCARE

SALLY OLIVIA KIM

FOREWORD BY TESS MAURICIO, MD, FAAD

The Countryman Press
A division of W. W. Norton & Company
Independent Publishers Since 1923

IMPORTANT NOTE

This volume is intended for use by healthy adults as a general information resource only. It is not a substitute for medical advice. Readers who are pregnant, nursing, or considering pregnancy, and readers who have been diagnosed with, or suspect they may have, any medical or psychological condition, should consult a licensed physician or other professional healthcare provider before introducing collagen to their diets.

Do not give collagen to infants or children. Do not use collagen to prevent or treat illness. Read manufacturers' labels carefully and avoid any product that contains ingredients to which you may be allergic or sensitive. The author and the publisher specifically disclaim responsibility for any adverse effects or consequences resulting from the use of this volume.

The Collagen Glow reflects the author's personal research and experience. Neither the author nor the publisher is engaged in rendering medical or other professional advice, and neither makes any representation or warranty with respect to the accuracy, completeness, or fitness for any particular purpose of the information herein. Specific results mentioned in this book not be typical.

Web addresses, if any, included in this book reflect links existing as of the date of first publication. The publisher is not responsible for the content of any website, blog, or information page other than its own.

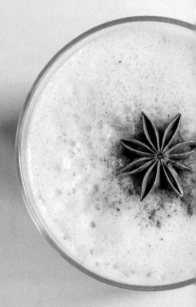

Text copyright © 2018 by Sally Olivia Kim
Foreword copyright © 2018 by
Tess Mauricio, MD, FAAD
Photographs copyright © 2018 by Jo Harding

For information about permission to reproduce selections from this book, write to Permissions, The Countryman Press, 500 Fifth Avenue, New York, NY 10110

For information about special discounts for bulk purchases, please contact W. W. Norton Special Sales at specialsales@wwnorton.com or 800-233-4830

Manufacturing by Versa Press
Book design by Nick Caruso Design
Photo styling by Brigitte Kozena
Production manager: Devon Zahn

The Countryman Press
www.countrymanpress.com

A division of W. W. Norton & Company, Inc.
500 Fifth Avenue, New York, NY 10110
www.wwnorton.com

Library of Congress
Cataloging-in-Publication Data

Names: Kim, Sally Olivia, author. | Mauricio, Tess, writer of foreword.
Title: The collagen glow : a guide to ingestible skincare / Sally Olivia Kim; foreword by Tess Mauricio, MD, FAAD.
Description: New York, NY : The Countryman Press, [2018] | Includes bibliographical references and index.
Identifiers: LCCN 2018031264
Subjects: LCSH: Skin—Care and hygiene. | Collagen—Therapeutic use. | Beauty, Personal.
Classification: LCC RL87 .K54 2018 | DDC 646.7/26—dc23 LC record available at https://lccn.loc.gov/2018031264

10 9 8 7 6 5 4 3 2 1

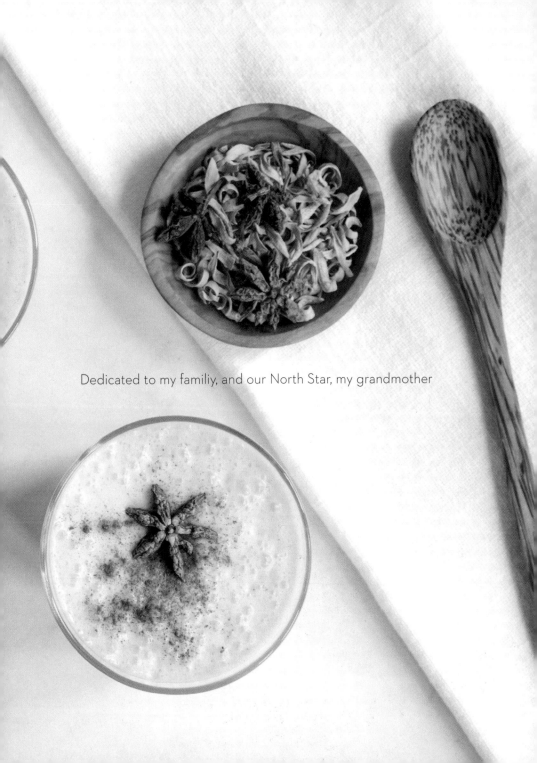

Dedicated to my familiy, and our North Star, my grandmother

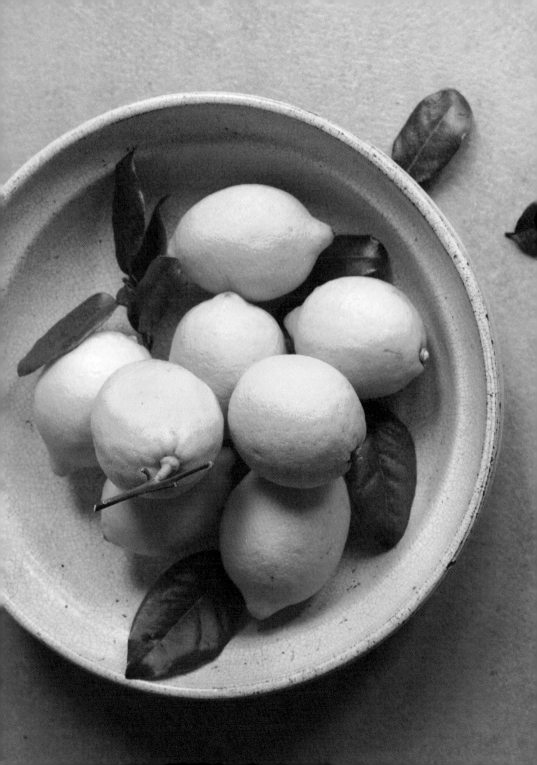

AUTHOR'S NOTE

I wrote this book because I truly believe that taking collagen has totally rejuvenated my skin and made me feel better all around. But not surprisingly, there are disagreements among doctors and others about the benefits and risks of ingesting collagen. Not everyone thinks it will have any effect, some caution about overdoing it, and others say it has some risks. Also, I can't promise that collagen will do for you what I think it has done for me: I don't know how old you are, what your skin looks like, what your regular diet is, or what kind of lifestyle you have; and I don't know whether you have any genetic or medical conditions or allergies that would make ingesting collagen inadvisable for you. So:

- Consult your doctor before you start to take collagen, especially if you are pregnant or nursing, or if you suffer from any allergy or other medical condition, and especially if you are taking any medication.

- Check the ingredients of whatever collagen powder you are considering using. The FDA doesn't regulate collagen supplements. Some collagen comes from shellfish, and many collagen powders contain eggs, to which some people are allergic.

- Check with your doctor before you start to include any new fruit, vegetable, or any other ingredient from my recipes as a regular part of your diet. Some foods carry risks for some people. For example, goji berries, which I use in one of my collagen shakes, can negatively interact with warfarin and diabetes drugs; and, even though, like most Koreans, I've been eating kimchi all my life, there is a dispute about whether kimchi causes stomach cancer. Even seemingly ordinary foods like pomegranates may be problematic for some people!

- Definitely consult your doctor if you have begun to ingest collagen regularly and you don't feel well. While there may be absolutely no connection, better to be safe than sorry.

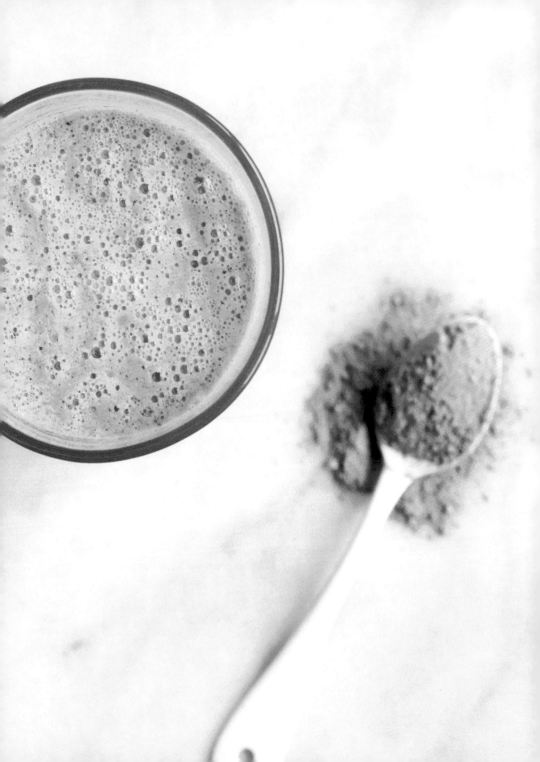

CONTENTS

FOREWORD BY
TESS MAURICIO, MD, FAAD*

When I was asked to write the foreword to Sally Kim's book, *The Collagen Glow*, I was thrilled for many reasons. Most important, Sally shares my belief that nutrition is the key to health. I am in my late forties now and I certainly have observed through experience and my own research that nutrition is key to health and beauty. In fact, I am probably one of the first dermatologists to talk to my fellow doctors and patients about nutrition and supplements because as we know we can effectively apply antioxidants, botanicals, and vitamins on our skin topically, and we can also provide our skin with the building blocks it needs by ingesting key ingredients through our diet and proper supplementation.

My interest in supplementation started with my husband's health journey and recovery from a brain tumor. His tumor was treated with chemotherapy but the experience sparked a passion for brain health and how to approach it holistically. We put our Stanford MD brains together, used our biochemistry and molecular biophysics education, and did our research on essential ingredients for brain health. In the process, we became believers that food has to be thought of as a means to deliver the parts and pieces, the biomolecules that are necessary for protein synthesis, energy production for maintenance, repair, and regeneration.

I believe there is absolutely something to be said about Sally's being Korean. My husband is Korean American and truthfully, one of the qualities I loved about him from the beginning was his beautiful skin! And as Sally explains, her grandmother's recipes for beauty truly involved recipes for food! Koreans (just like my fellow Filipinos and other Asian cultures) incorporate varying and rich sources of collagen in their native dishes, which were historically born out of necessity and poverty. Most Korean soup bases are broths made from boiling bones and marrow for hours—without the cooks usually thinking about the fact that these are all great sources of collagen. I believe that years of regular ingestion of collagen-rich foods, such as these, naturally increase the levels of biopeptides and amino acids that

---

* Publisher's note: Dr. Mauricio is a co-founder of Liveli, a nutritional supplement company

circulate in the bloodstream and, just like in the studies, end up concentrated in the dermis for days after eating the meal! So no wonder Sally found her grandmother's recipes healing not only in a spiritual sense but also on a biochemical and biomolecular level. She uses her culture and background to highlight the intrinsic beauty and skin benefits of a Korean diet. Not all of us have grandmas who can cook these amazing soups and dishes for us, but with today's technology, we can all have access to ingestible collagen, ingestible precursors to essential components to our skin's health and beauty. Throughout her book, Sally shows us an innovative, modern, and unconventional way to achieve our best! Who doesn't love food, recipes, and cookbooks?

The skin is the largest organ of the body, and as a dermatologist I am fully aware that it also has the most psychological impact to our overall well-being. Our skin is made up of the epidermis: the outermost layer; and the dermis: the innermost layer. Although what our eyes see is the epidermis, the dermis is where it all begins. Collagen plays a huge role in the health of this crucial layer. The structure of the dermis, the collagen, must be maintained so as to provide the proper structural support to the epidermis and allow the skin to function normally and appear healthy and youthful.

Speaking of optimization and dare I say it, biohacking, I am all for it. I love the results of optimizing my mind, body, and soul, and I love that when I tell people how old I am, they are usually shocked. Sally was amazed when I sent her my twentieth wedding anniversary family photo. Of course, I attribute some of my youthful looks to the cutting-edge cosmetic dermatology and regenerative aesthetic procedures now available in my clinics, which I take advantage of. But I also get this a lot: "Of course you look young, you are Asian!"

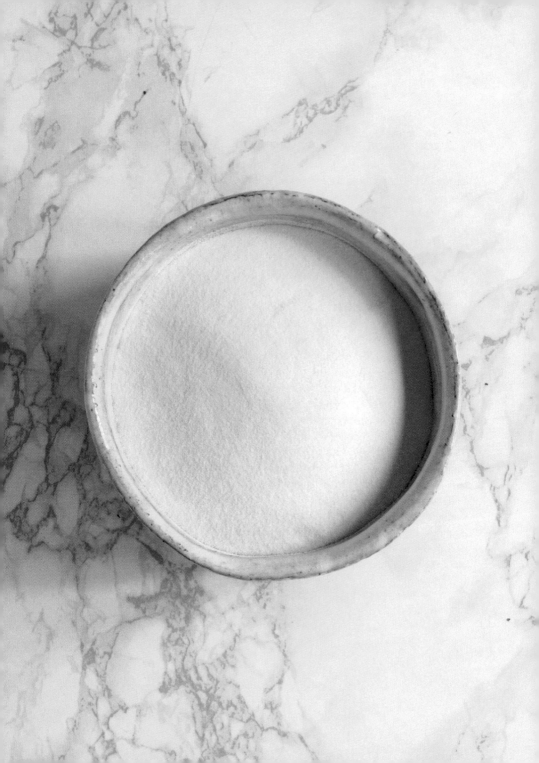

You don't have to be a genius to figure out that what you put into your body directly translates into how you look and feel. But despite knowing this all my life, I admit that I didn't realize just how true this was until I seriously burned myself in a cooking accident. That incident led me to initiate a deep dive into finding a cure—spoiler alert: it turned out to be ingesting collagen—turned me into something of a true believer on this topic. I also figured out that my Korean grandmother, my *halmuni*, with her bone broths and fish dinners, had been right all along about the importance of collagen for a healthy skin and body.

After my accident, I tried to fix the burns from the outside in. I bought every lotion, patch, and prescription ointment I could find. Nothing worked. I kept at it, researching everything I could find about skin, and how to heal and regenerate it as quickly as possible. I discovered a treatment using the skin of fish. Researchers in Brazil determined that tilapia contains a very high level of collagen proteins, and that by placing the fish skin directly onto the burned area, the collagen helped relieve pain and showed signs of helping to prevent scarring. Could this be the answer? Of course, I wasn't going to put fish skin all over my body, and I was already past the point of preventing initial scars. I decided to start taking collagen supplements, just to see what would happen. Less than a month of consuming 20 grams of collagen a day, I saw incredible changes. I have to add here that what I took is twice the recommended dose, so I'm not telling you to reproduce this experiment! But it did work for me. Not only were the burns on my arms starting to fade, but everywhere from head to toe, even my nails and hair, had started to look better. Everyone began asking me what eye cream I was using—and that's when I realized that ingesting collagen was making my skin the healthiest it had ever been since I was a kid, back when I was enjoying my grandmother's traditional cooking. She served every meal with a basket of roasted seaweed, grilled mackerel with its skin on, and a bowl of piping hot soup with bone broth as its base (chicken, pork, beef, or anchovy stock). And what all these dishes have in common is that they are all loaded with collagen, or as my grandmother calls it, *the good stuff.*

There's so much collagen in these side dishes and soups that after you're finished with a typical Korean meal, even your lips get taut and sticky (a sign of your skin's becoming more revitalized)!

Why is that important? Because collagen is a type of protein that all living, breathing animals—including humans—produce. It makes up our bones, muscles, skin, and hair. It's also the most abundant protein in our body that holds our bones, muscles, and especially skin, together (collagen comprises 70 percent of the protein found in skin). Collagen plays an integral role in keeping our skin plump and youthful, as it is key in our body's facilitation of new regeneration of skin, muscle, bone, and joint cells. Yet unfortunately, as we age, our body's ability to produce our much needed supply of collagen diminishes at a rate of 1 percent per year, resulting in the depletion of collagen in our skin cells. Consequently, our skin fails to retain moisture as it once used to, leading to less hydrated cells and looser, weaker, stretchier, and thinner skin (and of course, this is what causes wrinkles, fine lines, dry skin, cellulite, and even brittle hair).

Despite religiously yet unknowingly consuming collagen all my life—I didn't always put two and two together—I always attributed my skin to "Korean genetics," the same way everyone else did. Because, to be honest, I didn't really ever *do* anything to my skin. I was terrible at making a daily habit of those expensive products that I'd purchase on a whim, and in comparison to my friends who were getting regular facials and peels, my skincare efforts were minimal.

My family moved to the States when I was ten years old, so my diet changed at that time (as did my skin). But once I started back on collagen—this time, in powdered form—not only did my burns heal, but the differences I noticed were not just on my arms, but in my face and hair. My eyelashes, brows, and hair got so much thicker, and my skin no longer just looked great—according to my friends, it looked "Photoshopped," "glowy," and "as soft as a baby's bottom."

Even my number-one skin problems—dry skin and enlarged pores—seemed to have disappeared without my even knowing, over the course of my collagen regimen.

It truly felt like a miracle, but was one that was literally hard to swallow. I was using unflavored powdered bovine collagen, which was designed to be mixed into drinks; coffee was the most popular as it was supposed to mask the taste of the collagen. Even in the blackest of the coffees, though, I was able to pick up on the earthy, musty, icky flavor. I actually ended up just mixing my dose of collagen into a bit of water, holding my nose, and gulping it down. The fact is, there are people who are able to stand the strong taste of bovine collagen; I was not one of them.

But, knowing how beneficial collagen was for me from head to toe, I kept at it. I started telling everyone I knew about this wonder supplement and got quite a few people started on it. The taste continued to be an issue. To me, it was a challenge. And after months of research, tasting essentially every collagen brand out there, and then flavoring it with other, delicious superfoods, I found the king of all collagens, one that would work with the other superfood powders I liked to add.

I happily sent it out to every single one of my friends and family. But despite their approval, I came across other obstacles: they kept forgetting to take it daily; plus, some of the plastic tubs were a hassle to open and they'd lose the measuring spoon. Without taking it every day, they did not see the results that I was seeing.

So, I decided to reverse-engineer the experience a bit; if people genuinely liked the taste of the collagen drink and looked forward to drinking it, then they wouldn't think of it as medicine, but like any other flavored beverage out there. On a mission to get them hooked, and with the goal that my final product would taste *good* (so good that you'd have no idea that there were 10 grams of fish skin in it), I started formulating, and invented hundreds of recipes with collagen in them.

Finally, when my friends and family couldn't taste the difference between the matcha latte that had the collagen in it and the one without, that's when I knew that I had succeeded. And that's the start of my ingestible beauty brand, Crushed Tonic, and the purpose of this book, and this collection of recipes—to show you that collagen, if prepared well, could be something you enjoy, and even love.

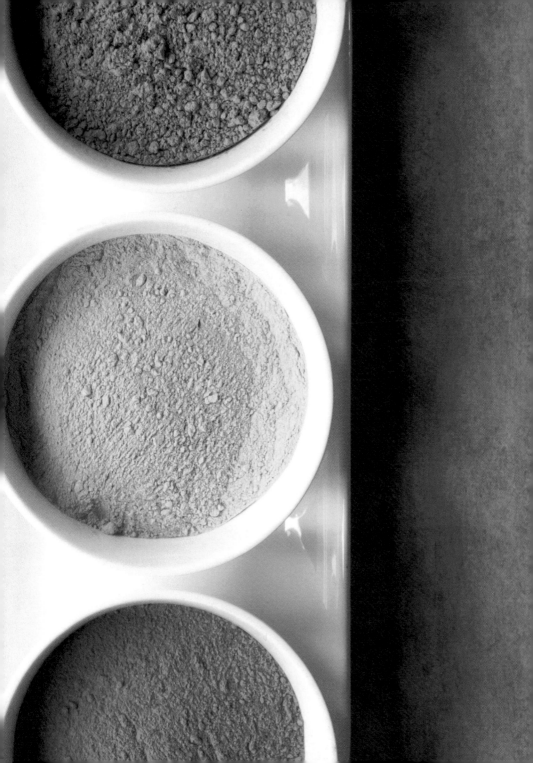

Collagen 101

It can be confusing to decipher what collagen is, especially when there are so many different terms to describe it: collagen peptides, hydrolyzed collagen, gelatin collagen, collagen type I, type II, type III—list goes on. And then there are all of the different sources: cows, fish? What about pills, liquid, or powder?

In this book, I will help you answer some of those questions, share with you my personal journey with collagen, and offer 40 recipes that can help make ingesting collagen an easy, delicious, and daily routine.

WHAT IS COLLAGEN?

Mainstream usage of collagen has been mostly topical, which leads people to mistakenly believe it to be only something to apply externally to skin (and in some cases, inject with a needle to plump the skin).

Collagen is a natural protein that our body produces. It is a major structural component of the human body (different types of collagen make up our skin, bones, muscles, and joints), and we depend on collagen to keep our skin plump, hair strong, bones healthy, joints lubricated, and digestive system working smoothly.

And though our body is able to produce ample amounts of collagen when we are young, unfortunately, sometime after the age of twenty-five, our bodily production of collagen begins to decline at a rate of 1.5 percent per year (in addition to the decline in the quality of our produced collagen). By our mid-forties, our collagen levels may have fallen by as much as 30 percent. Without collagen, our cells lose structure, increasingly becoming weaker, stretchier, and thinner—and essentially, this decline is the true cause of many of our skin woes, such as wrinkles, fine lines, dark circles, dry skin, and cellulite.

But don't worry; you can make up for the collagen you lose by consuming collagen, the foundation of healthy skin.

TYPES OF COLLAGENS

Collagen occurs in many places throughout the body, making up a huge 90 percent of our bone mass and 30 percent of all other proteins our body produces. There are various types of collagen (at least 16), each type being found in different areas of the body: the skin, connective tissues, lungs, muscles, joints, blood cells, arteries, and more.

The six most common types are:

COLLAGEN TYPE I

- Found in our skin, tendons, ligaments, and heart
- Crucial for healing wounds and holding together our muscles and bones, in addition to making our tissue strong so it doesn't tear

COLLAGEN TYPE II

- Found in our cartilage and connective tissues
- Because our joints rely on well-lubricated cartilage, collagen is integral in optimizing our joint health.

COLLAGEN TYPE III

- Found in our organs, such as our heart and skin (alongside type I)
- The reticulate in type III helps give our skin and tissue their elasticity and firmness.

COLLAGEN TYPE IV

- Integral in lining our digestive and respiratory organs

COLLAGEN TYPE V

- Supports new hair formation as well as placentas

COLLAGEN TYPE X

- Important to the formation of new bone

If this sounds confusing, think about it this way: if you divided your body into 16 different sections, there would be some type of collagen in every single quadrant, and multiple types of collagen in varying quadrants. Type I and type III collagen would be in every section, because your skin covers your entire body—and hence these are considered to be the most abundant types of collagen.

WHAT KIND OF BENEFITS CAN I HOPE TO SEE?

First and foremost, daily consumption of collagen, which you now know is found in almost every part of your body, may dramatically improve your skin.

In various studies, survey respondents noted improvements in their skin in as little as four to eight weeks.

And although I emphasize the benefits of collagen to skin for most of this book, when you ingest collagen, it seems the benefits spread to the rest of your body, too, from head to toe.

But before I get into these benefits, I'd like to talk about the makeup of collagen—the reason that collagen is so beneficial to us.

AMINO ACIDS

Some of the most confusing bits of the science behind collagen have to do with amino acids. Amino acids are crucial building blocks of our body. A large proportion of our cells, muscles, and tissue is made up of amino acids, and they carry out many important bodily functions, such as giving cells their structure. We depend on amino acids—they are at the basis of all life processes, and insufficiency can lead to negative impacts on our skin, hair, bones, and health (arthritis and osteoporosis; high cholesterol; diabetes; obesity; hair loss; poor sleep, mood, and performance, and even virility).

There are 20 different amino acids in the human body. These can be grouped into three different categories—essential, semiessential, and nonessential. (Note: The use of the terms *essential* and *nonessential* is not to indicate one is less essential for our health than the other—it just indicates whether the human body can create those amino acids on its own.)

ESSENTIAL AMINO ACIDS

There are eight amino acids that our bodies need but cannot produce, so we have to eat foods that contain them.

- isoleucine
- leucine
- lysine
- methionine
- phenylalanine
- threonine
- tryptophan
- valine

SEMIESSENTIAL AMINO ACIDS

There are two semiessential amino acids that our bodies need but cannot produce, so we have to eat foods that contain them as well.

- arginine
- histidine

NONESSENTIAL AMINO ACIDS

Those are 10 nonessential amino acids found in our body. We *can* produce these acids on our own, but ingesting them from external sources will still be beneficial in supporting our day-to-day functions:

- alanine
- asparagine
- aspartic acid
- cysteine
- glutamic acid
- glutamine
- glycine
- proline
- serin
- tyrosine

Collagen, as a complex protein, contains 18 out of the 20 existing amino acids found in our body. And studies have shown that these 18 amino acids, when ingested, support all of the different various functions of our body in different ways: our skin, hair, brain, bones, teeth, nails, heart, digestion, muscles, weight, mood, virility, and even sleep.

HOW CAN WE CONSUME COLLAGEN?

For us to consume collagen, we must look to high-protein parts of animals.

You're probably thinking, "Oh, I eat chicken every day—I'm fine."

But here's the catch. Collagen is not in a salmon fillet or a piece of chicken breast—but in the animals' skin, joints, bones, and muscle tissue.

Collagen Helps . . .

- Skin
- Hair and nails
- Joints
- Bones and teeth
- Muscle tissues, ligaments, and tendons
- Digestion
- Lower stress and anxiety

WHAT IF I DON'T WANT TO BE EATING ANIMALS' BONES OR SKIN?
Americans do not generally eat these parts of animals (and now
you're thinking, *Other countries eat these parts?* And the answer is
yes—chicken feet are a delicacy in Korean cuisine, among others).

The Korean diet is full of collagen for many reasons, but an interest-
ing one that my grandmother would never let me forget is that Korea
used to be an extremely poor country. Although Korea, and where I
grew up in Seoul, is so developed that it mirrors the ever-cosmopolitan
New York City, even just 50 years ago it was thought to be a third-world
country. When my grandmother told me she grew up in a straw-hut
house, I remember I didn't believe her. So when I wouldn't finish my
food, she would always tell me a story about the importance of food:
when my grandma was younger, food was so scarce, she could barely
ever have meat—and it was considered to be the biggest luxury when
she *was* able to get it for her children. And because it was such a rarity
to have chicken at the table, when she was able to get it, she would
split it seven different ways for her five children, my grandfather, and
herself—and she did not discriminate as to which part of the animal they
got. This explains why Koreans leave zero waste of anything—they had
to make do with the little they were given—hence the creation of such
foods as fried chicken feet. But interestingly enough, it happens to be
that Koreans had accidentally cracked the code!

The closest Americans get to eating collagen in its natural state is as bone broth—which can be made by simmering bones (or backs, necks, and feet) for more than 12 hours, until a rich and almost sticky broth is produced.

Bone Broth

Essentially, bone broth is cooked collagen. And all the benefits that are touted for bone broth are simply benefits derived from the collagen—specifically, from ingesting amino acids in the collagen.

SO, DO I HAVE TO MAKE BONE BROTH EVERY DAY TO GET MY COLLAGEN?
Not at all.

We don't need to turn to the onerous labor of cooking bone broth to get our collagen.

Personally, I'm not the biggest proponent of daily consumption of bone broth, anyway: there may not be enough collagen in the serving you are having, and if you are cooking the bone broth with lots of salt and seasonings, it will probably be incredibly high in sodium.

For those of us who want to avoid sodium, don't have time to be cooking cauldrons of bone broth daily, or have zero desire to munch on 10 grams of raw fish skin or bones, no need to worry: collagen peptides are the answer.

I KEEP HEARING ABOUT COLLAGEN GELATIN. HOW IS IT DIFFERENT FROM COLLAGEN PEPTIDES?
Collagen gelatin is usually in a brittle, flat, almost papery form, and when mixed with water, turns into more of a gel, whereas collagen peptides are like protein powder and turn into liquid without much texture.

Gelatin and collagen peptides have the same amino acid profile (18 amino acids, of which eight are considered to be essential amino acids), and an identical source (skin, bones, tissue).

Gelatin is often used in recipes as thickeners—it is what gives food a lot of its creamy texture. Collagen peptides, on the other hand, when dissolved perfectly, do not change the consistency of beverages or foods.

The chemical difference between them is that gelatin only goes through partial hydrolysis, whereas collagen peptides go through a more aggressive one. Peptides are easier than gelatin for your body to digest and absorb, which means the amino acids in collagen peptides, also known as hydrolyzed collagen, may be more bioavailable and therefore more effective.

WHAT IS HYDROLYSIS?

Hydrolysis is a fancy word to describe the process of breaking something down with water. Our body cannot utilize collagen in its native state (as the skin, bones, or connective tissue of animals). For this reason, companies that make collagen powder put the collagen compounds through an intense process called hydrolysis, whereby these large sources of edible collagen are cooked, boiled, and then hydrolyzed.

Hydrolyzed collagen peptides have a more than 90 percent absorption rate, three times higher than when their collagen source is ingested directly from food.

HOW CAN I TAKE COLLAGEN PEPTIDES?

Collagen peptides are offered in a variety of forms: collagen pills vs. liquid vs. powder.

LIQUID COLLAGEN: A ready-to-consume product that comes in an 8- to 32-ounce bottle. Its collagen is in a base of water and often includes flavors to make it tastier, and you will have to consume it by taking the amount the manufacturer recommends on the bottle. The liquid collagen will save you the time of mixing collagen powders yourself.

COLLAGEN POWDER: Collagen peptides in their most raw form are a fine powder. This powder is usually mixed with water, creating liquid collagen (which is by far the most beneficial for the body as it is absorbed most efficiently). The key to assessing collagen powder is through its taste, purity, and color. Not all collagen powders are created equal, and to find a high-quality collagen powder that you can take every day, you should try a few different ones and see which you like best—both in taste and in ease of use.

COLLAGEN TABLETS: Generally one capsule or tablet provides 1 gram of collagen (equal to 1,000 mg). Follow the manufacturer's directions to determine how many capsules/tablets should be taken daily.

COLLAGEN CANDIES, GUMMIES, AND CHOCOLATES: There are candy alternatives for collagen—however, they are usually made with high-fructose corn syrup or other artificial sweeteners. Collagen gummy bears are often made with gelatin.

I prefer powders over tablets, capsules, gummies, and liquids, as I hate the feeling and experience of swallowing pills (and to swallow 10? No, thank you!). But whether it be in liquid, powder, capsule, or candy form, its essence is all the same: collagen peptides. However you consume your collagen, I have found that the most important thing is to take your collagen daily, and for at least four weeks straight, assuming you are tolerating it well.

WHERE ARE COLLAGEN PEPTIDES SOURCED FROM?

MARINE (A.K.A. FISH) COLLAGEN

- Sourced from fish skin and scales
- Rich in type I collagen
- Rich in glycine, proline, and hydroxyproline

BOVINE (A.K.A. COW) COLLAGEN

- Sourced from cow hides, bones, and muscles
- Rich in type I and type III collagen
- Rich in glycine and proline
- Helps produce creatine, which is beneficial for building muscle

AVIARY (A.K.A. CHICKEN) COLLAGEN

- sourced from chicken bones, cartilage, and tissues
- contains type II collagen

PORCINE (A.K.A. PIG) COLLAGEN

- Sourced from pig skin

VEGETARIAN COLLAGEN

- Sourced from eggshells and egg whites
- Rich in type I, but also includes types II, IV, and X

Marine and bovine collagen both perform well in studies and get similar results, primarily because both are bioavailable and dissolve great in liquids.

For vegetarians and everyone else who consume eggs: egg whites are high in both lysine and proline, so adding more egg whites to your diet could help support your body's natural production of collagen. Collagen-like proteins have been found in the eggshell membranes of hens, as well. Vegetarian collagen comes from chicken egg whites and eggshells, which offers types I and V collagen (type V is found in relatively minimal amounts, in hair and placenta mostly, so it's not one you need to focus on, but doesn't hurt to consume it if you prefer vegetarian powders).

There is no direct source of consumable collagen for vegans, as collagen is an inherently animal product. Vegan collagen does exist, made from plants that are good for the skin. Many of those on the market include extra vitamins and minerals. The downside is that they may also contain sugars, dextrose compounds, and even preservatives or fillers.

Vegans (and even those who are able to take animal-derived collagen) have still other ways to help their body's collagen levels flourish: one is by eating foods that help stimulate the body's production of the vital protein. Another is to consume plant foods that are packed with hyaluronic acid, a naturally occurring acid found in the human body that acts as a lubrication agent for our hair and skin. Hyaluronic acid has properties similar to those of animal collagen, and plays a critical role in skin health, with its remarkable ability to bind to 1,000 times its weight in moisture. My favorite source of hyaluronic acid is seaweed: Koreans eat roasted seaweed at almost every meal and I believe it to be a powerful superfood. Other hyaluronic acid and collagen production–stimulating foods include green vegetables for vitamin C; red vegetables, such as tomatoes, for lycopene; mushrooms; and nuts.

I suggest trying each type of collagen source and seeing which kind your body tells you it feels strongest on. Also, listen to your body and see which is the easiest on your stomach.

DOES IT MATTER WHAT TYPES OF COLLAGEN OR WHICH ANIMAL COLLAGEN SOURCE IT COMES FROM?

As I explained previously, there are different types of collagens in our body. And though some research suggests that consuming certain types to benefit the particular parts of the body (for example, types I and III if we want better hair, skin, and nails, vs. type II for cartilage and joints), most collagen experts and doctors don't see the necessity in consuming specific types for specific purposes. According to collagen expert Nick Bitz, a licensed, board-certified naturopathic doctor (N.D.) and chief science officer for a supplement company called YouTheory, "When you ingest collagen, you are ingesting amino acids that help rebuild all of your own collagen in the body. Not just Type

I or III, but every type." That is, when we ingest collagen, our body breaks it down into amino acids that are then absorbed, transported to cells, and used to make new collagen proteins suited for our body—new forms of collagen no longer corresponding directly to the type associated with their original source.

While many different types of collagen do exist—differentiated by where in the body it's sourced and its amino acid structure, and there can be benefits that arise from ingesting heavier concentrations of certain amino acids in those different types of collagen, most collagens have a similar amino acid profile, and Dr. Bitz at YouTheory explains, they're all still the same protein.

I'M SOLD ON THE BENEFITS. BUT IS COLLAGEN SAFE TO INGEST? WHAT ABOUT SIDE EFFECTS?

Technically, collagen is really just like any other protein you are consuming on your plate—something you've been eating here and there all your life (yet probably had no idea).

And even if taking collagen powder may *seem* like a foreign concept, it's been around for decades, and has been used in Asian and European countries for quite some time.

Still, as with everything we put into our body, we must know where exactly a substance originated from, and how it was processed. Like many protein powders on the market today, collagen powder *can* contain things that are toxic for the body—metals, pollutants, contaminants, and more. Luckily, the standards for making collagen powder have been raised significantly in the last few years, and with the help of the Internet, we can find out quickly what goes in the collagen we are purchasing. If a company cannot trace its collagen every step of the way back to when it was in its original form, I'd stay far away from that brand. Properly processed collagen would have been first sourced from non-GMO fish, cow, chicken, or pork; then purified; then hydrolyzed in an enzymatic solution; then filtered; then milled into powder, which is again sterilized; and then spray dried.

Aside from the physical source of the collagen, you need to look at the broader picture: you should know where the source itself came from (just as you should know where your salmon or steak came from). For example, if it's marine collagen, is it from fish from clean waters or waters contaminated with heavy metals or radiation?

Is it from fish that are generally higher in mercury? If it's bovine or aviary collagen, then is the source from grass-fed beef, naturally raised chickens, or other farm animals sustainably raised in every possible good manner? Or is it from commercially raised cattle, poultry, and so on?

Hydrolyzed collagen is the most bioavailable, which means your body is more likely to be able to absorb its nutrients without reacting to it negatively.

I am not a doctor, so I can only speak for it personally, but I have been taking and recommending collagen to my friends and family for years, and no one has ever reported any side effects—even my vegan friends who haven't consumed animal product for years don't react to the collagen.

Having said that, collagen in bigger forms, such as gelatin or in its source's natural state, could be too big for our body to break down, which then could cause digestive problems, such as gas and bloating—which is why I'd recommend always turning to collagen peptides over anything else. Because I am not a doctor, I want to remind you that it's important for you to speak with a physician before making any changes in your diet if you are suffering from any health condition or if you are nursing a baby, pregnant, or planning to become pregnant. Even if you do not suffer from any health condition and are neither pregnant nor nursing, it's important to understand that there may be risks associated with ingesting particular kinds of collagen, or collagen from particular sources. For example, Livestrong says that collagen from marine sources contains a lot of calcium. If that calcium raises your overall calcium levels by too much, you may experience "constipation, bone pain, fatigue, nausea, vomiting, and abnormal heart rhythms." You also may experience allergic reactions and have a bad taste in your mouth.

HOW DO I KNOW THAT MY COLLAGEN IS OF HIGH QUALITY?
To test the quality of your collagen powder, simply pour a little bit of lukewarm water into a glass or a cup, put a scoop of collagen into it, and mix it until the powder begins to dissolve.

With high-quality, pure collagen, you will see that the color of the water will stay translucent. In an interview with Well+Good, Naomi Whittel, a supplements entrepreneur who has been studying collagen for the past 20 years, advises to "steer clear of anything yellow, brown, or another tinted color—that's one way to spot less-than-premium quality." If you're buying a collagen in powder form, Whittel says it should be colorless (when mixed with water) and tasteless. "This shows how pure it is."

And of course, we must always pay attention to the label, and check the origin of the collagen—according to YouTheory's naturopath, Dr. Bitz, country origins matter: "Collagen sourced from China is really cheap and just not up to the standards of higher-quality stuff," he says. And because supplements are actually *unable* to be regulated by the FDA, brands should make sure to turn to quality manufacturers and suppliers that sourced only the most premium, high-quality ingredients (and they should be able to trace every step of the way back to where their collagen comes from).

Tip: Read reviews, and make sure you test a few before really ritualizing one brand.

HOW ABOUT FOR PREGNANT WOMEN?

If you are pregnant or breastfeeding, or if you are planning to become pregnant in the near future, you should always ask your doctor before you start to ingest collagen.

HOW MUCH IS THE RIGHT AMOUNT?

This will always be up for a debate.

Many brands recommend a minimum of 8 to 10 grams of hydrolyzed collagen. Other sources suggest that 6 to 10 grams daily is the appropriate dose.

Most powders come with a scoop that's about 10 grams—some brands recommend one scoop; some, two scoops. Then there are the powders that come premeasured, in handy packets (perhaps beautifully designed, like Crushed Tonic!), which contain about 10 grams per packet. Always check the manufacturer's recommendation and do not exceed the recommended dose.

WHEN SHOULD I TAKE COLLAGEN?

The best time to take collagen is when there's nothing in your stomach. This could be in the morning when you first wake up, before bed, or a few hours after eating a meal. It's important to bypass the digestive process when taking collagen supplements. You want the collagen to be in your bloodstream in its present form, not digested by stomach acid or mixed in with your food for breakdown during digestion.

SHOULD I TAKE ANYTHING ELSE ALONG WITH COLLAGEN?
VITAMIN C: According to the Linus Pauling Institute researchers at Oregon State University, vitamin C has a distinct role in collagen synthesis: without vitamin C, our body is slower in healing wounds and producing collagen. Thus, it makes sense to have some vitamin C added to your collagen supplement. I also like to have a clementine or orange in the morning to spike up my collagen production.

PROBIOTICS: Probiotics are one of the latest ingredients added to collagen supplements. High-quality probiotics are known to do a lot—and because our stomach, a.k.a. the second brain, is the ruler of our overall health, we need to do all things possible to keep it happy. Because when our stomach is off, our skin takes a beating almost immediately!

HYALURONIC ACID: Hyaluronic acid (HA) is a substance known to improve skin hydration from both the inside and out. HA has been shown to have a durable effect to retain moisture in the skin from inside the body. In a month-long study, surveyed individuals who added hyaluronic acid to their diet showed significant reductions in skin dryness and wrinkles, and improvements in skin moisture and fullness. It also doubles as a powerful moisturizer: it can attract around 1,000 times its own weight in water—a feature that few other compounds have. Its ability to retain so much moisture is why hyaluronic acid is so popular in skincare products. The compound also plays key roles throughout our body: it lubricates joints, helps provide moisture, and ensures our eyes don't dry out. And last but not least, it also helps decrease collagen loss in our body! I often refer to it as unicorn blood, as it is a clear, viscous, Jell-O–like gel that works magic on my skin.

SUPERFOODS: Superfoods are often added to collagen powders to provide flavoring and other health benefits. I've selected matcha, turmeric, and lucuma as the superfood flavorings to my formula.

Because matcha induces a sense of calm while simultaneously boosting your energy, concentration, memory, and metabolism, it can keep you full and awake for hours.

WHAT SHOULD I NOT TAKE WITH COLLAGEN?

The main rule of what not to take with collagen is foods that are eaten in a meal.

Anything that requires digestion is a no-no because it will interfere with the absorption of collagen into the bloodstream (also see the discussion of charcoal, page 118).

I also recommend forgoing collagen blends that contain added sugars as well as other preservatives and chemical additives—a lot of brands, to mask the taste, have been formulated with artificial flavors—which indeed defeat the whole purpose of their being healthy!

I GET THAT THE POWDER IS EASIER, BUT WOULDN'T IT BE BETTER FOR ME TO GET THE COLLAGEN FROM WHOLE FOODS?

Often, when we prepare some of these collagen-rich foods (of course, every meal prep is different), we usually cook them with a lot of things that aren't quite so great for you, such as salt, and then packed with preservatives that are often carcinogenic (such as fried fish or chicken wings). And when one consumes fish skin, which is where we source collagen from primarily, it is usually deep-fried, or loaded with sodium.

Hence, we can't advise you to eat 10 whole grams of fish skin too often, let alone every day (and the daily aspect can't be emphasized more, as our body cannot store protein for longer than 24 hours).

What Are Probiotics?

Probiotics are live cultures that help balance the good and bad bacteria in our gut. By supporting the excretion of radical toxins from our systems, probiotics help our skin become stronger, happier, and healthier. Probiotics can help fight gut inflammation, help the body absorb certain types of nutrients, and keep the immune system in optimum shape. They may also help alleviate allergic and inflammatory skin disorders by increasing our immunity and optimizing digestion.

And how do these little probiotic soldiers help our skin? What probiotics do for our health and our skin, is almost immeasurable: our stomach, a.k.a. the second brain, is actually the ruler of our overall health. With probiotics, our stomach achieves that needed homeostasis much more easily. And they help fend off a lot of what causes problems, and by their supporting our body's excretion process of pushing the radical toxins that make our skin problematic, out of our system, our skin becomes stronger, happier, and healthier. This was something my grandmother would never let me forget if I ever decided to avoid eating kimchi at lunch.

IS COLLAGEN GLUTEN-FREE? DAIRY-FREE? IS IT PALEO-FRIENDLY?

Collagen powder, by itself, should be gluten-free, dairy-free, sugar-free . . . free of everything *but* animal skin and bones or vegetarian-sourced substances, such as seaweed. Many brands are certified kosher. If you are allergic to anything, you will want to know whether the collagen powder you are using was processed with any other substances. Even if it doesn't say that on the bottle, the bottle should identify the facility where the collagen was processed. You can contact that facility and ask whether the collagen was processed with other substances.

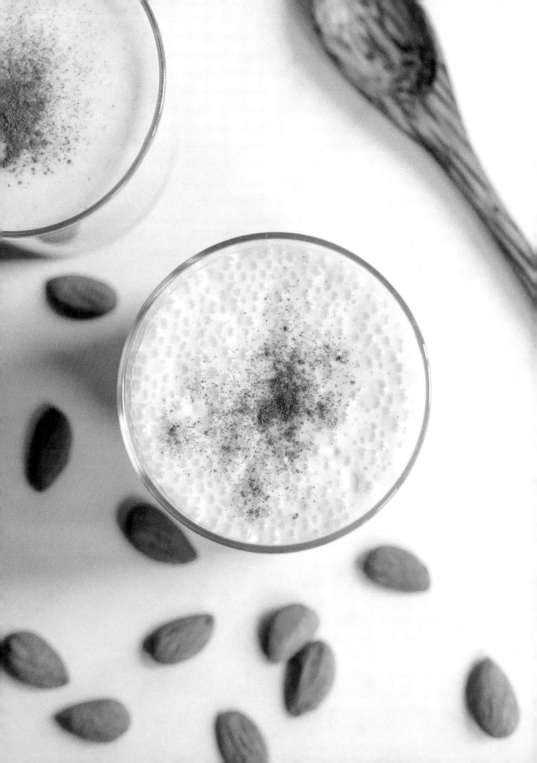

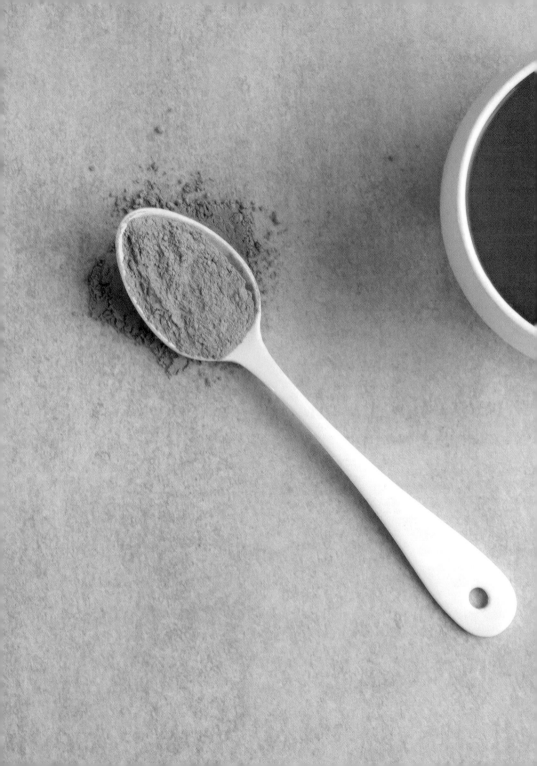

MY PERSONAL PREFERENCE

Because I get asked about my personal experience with collagen often—and because I've been asked the same questions so frequently, I figured I'd share them with you as well.

Q & A

What is your personal favorite type of collagen?

While founding Crushed Tonic, I made a conscious choice to use only marine collagen. From the research I've done, it tastes the best and is considered to be the most effective for skin (studies show that marine collagen might be absorbed more readily into the body because the protein peptides are smaller than those of cows).

37

How often do you take collagen? How much of it?

I take 10 grams every day, sometimes twice a day. But I do not suggest exceeding the dose recommended by the manufacturer of whatever collagen brand you are using.

Favorite recipe?

My favorite recipes are supersimple: the Matcha Tonic (page 48) and the Golden Milk Tumeric Latte (page 71) (hence the two being chosen as Crushed Tonic flavors). I also love making chocolate smoothie bowls!

How do I prepare my collagen lattes?

I don't like drinking lattes with any collagen clumps, but I also don't always have an electric whisk with me. So I hacked the process a little bit; now, all I need is an empty water bottle.

COLLAGEN 101

I'll pour my crush into an empty water bottle and then add a tiny bit of water (really, just 1 teaspoon. It's all about the proportions here, so don't add too much water).

I'll shake the bottle until the crush has dissolved and turned into an elixir.

Then, I heat coconut, almond, or pea milk (my favorite is pea milk) in a microwave for 1 to 2 minutes.

Finally, I'll add the collagen mixture to the heated latte mixture and stir. I sometimes like to add such things as vanilla extract, nondairy creamers, and superfood powders to spice things up a bit!

What benefits have you seen specifically?

Over the course of my two-years-plus collagen regimen, here are some of the things I've observed:

- I become fuller and more satiated throughout the day. This makes sense, because it's essentially like drinking bone broth, and since every drink is packed with 10 grams of protein, I don't get hungry for hours after.

- My hair grew so much more quickly, and my eyelashes and eyebrows grew in thicker. My anxiety had caused my hair to fall out (either that, or I tugged at it every five seconds), but after drinking collagen for six months–plus, my bald spot sprouted back up with hair! (Yes, a bald spot. I started to have one since the age of sixteen because I did cheerleading and dance all of my life, and the supercrisp, superhigh ponytails did a number on the root of my hair strands. It was so bad that sometimes my sister would add eyeshadow to color them in before my recitals).

- My skin is so much more hydrated. I used to have chronically dry skin that would peel (the *worst* over the winter months in New York City), so I always had a spritz and facial lotion with me, everywhere I went. I barely need to wear moisturizer now!
- My pores around my nose have gotten smaller.
- My under-eye dark circles have gone away. This truly was such a crazy discovery for me; I used to have purple rings underneath my eyes.
- I no longer need to wear foundation or cover up as much.
- My skin looks more dewy and glowing.
- My skin has gotten brighter, tighter, from head to toe: with less cellulite in my thighs.
- I've lost weight; again, it's just like drinking bone broth (one that's flavored with my favorite ingredients, and that tastes nothing like bone broth). So, not only did I never forget to drink it because I loved it so much, I consumed fewer calories throughout the day.

But beyond all these benefits, my favorite part is the ritual of making and drinking my Crushed Tonic/collagen latte every day. I wake up, and instead of running out the door to the next coffee shop, I start prepping my collagen latte. And I smile the entire time I'm drinking it! It's become such a habit that now my mornings feel incomplete without it—so when you do give it a try, I really recommend that you take five minutes to really prep and make your tonic the most perfect for you.

I love my collagen with a nut milk latte base. So, if you would like to have more of a milk base than water, make sure to mix the powder into a bit of water first, and add to the cup of your favorite milk!

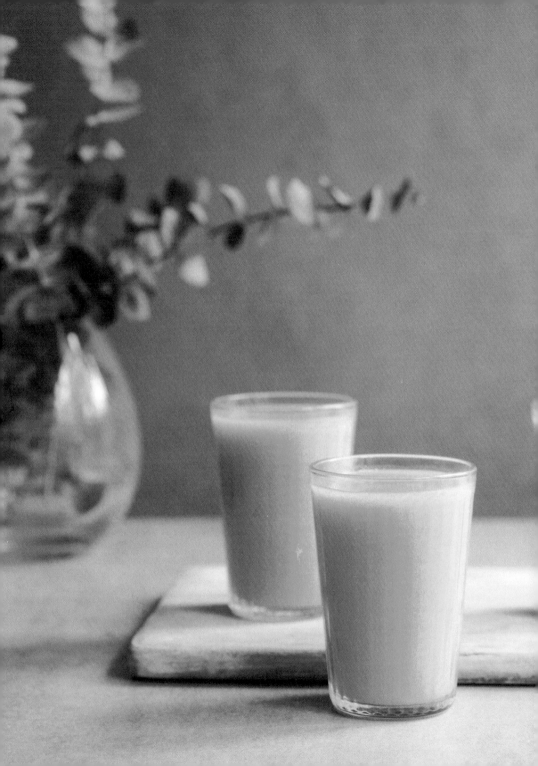

Hot and Cold Drinks

Now that you know which collagen works for you, and all the benefits you'll see, let's introduce you to the recipes that will help you integrate collagen into your daily routine and diet—recipes that will help you make it not just an easy habit, but an enjoyable one.

For best results, you should consume collagen daily, at least in the beginning of your regimen. Since our body cannot store protein the way we store our fats and sugars (and as with all types of proteins, our body's supply of it must be replenished daily), it's essential that we don't just do it here and there—but truly commit to it. (It is also worth noting that many collagen studies required participants to ingest collagen daily for one to three months, so we don't really *know* how taking collagen less frequently, or for a shorter period of time, would affect us.)

Since becoming hooked on it, I've developed dozens of recipes that make taking your collagen an easy and pleasurable task—and I want to share those recipes with you.

These drinks are similar in nutritive profile as the Korean meals I ate as a kid—collagen dense, gluten-free, low in sugar—and packed with other superfoods that are great for your skin, hair, and health. I guess mom was right after all!

Note: You might decide that liquid collagen or collagen pills make more sense for you; however, for the purpose of this cookbook, we will be using collagen in powdered form, as you can put it into just about anything and everything: water, coffees, juices, teas, smoothies, shakes, soups, cocktails, baked goods, candy—the options are truly limitless once you get the hang of it, and you wouldn't be changing the flavor of the drink or food at all!

TIPS & DIRECTIONS

I often say that to truly benefit from ingesting collagen, it's important to know how to take it. Here are some tips I've picked up along the way:

- If you are like me, you won't like drinking your collagen with any clumps (don't forget, at the end of the day, it is protein powder, which is best consumed when shaken up or blitzed). But because it's such fine protein powder, you can make do without an electric milk frother or juicer. Instead of directly mixing the powder into a big glass or bottle of liquid, pour a little bit (really, even just a sip) of lukewarm water into a container first, then add your collagen, and either shake or stir vigorously for about ten seconds. You'll end up with a very small amount of liquid collagen that can be easily mixed into just about everything.

- I love my collagen with a nut milk latte base. So, if you would like to have more of a milk base than a water base, make sure to mix the powder into a bit of water first, and then add to a hot cup of your favorite milk!

- I also love to make my lattes creamy, so I turn to denser milks, such as pea milk. If you're more of an almond milk type but want a thicker consistency, you can even turn to wholesome coffee creamer brands—adding even a tiny bit would make the latte richer and more decadent.

- Get creative. Mix it up. Some of my favorite drinks are a product of my accidentally combining two ingredients that would never go with each other (but look like the same thing). Teas are lovely to mix together. I love mixing Earl Grey tea with matcha, and rooibos tea with cacao. I even like getting creative with different flavors of nondairy milks. I love flavoring any base—whether it be almond, cashew, coconut, or soy—with nontraditional superelixirs, such as rose water or honeydew juice (blitzed-up honeydew).

- "Good for you" doesn't have to mean that it has to taste bad. And when it comes to smoothies, I am a proponent of not removing the sweet ingredients entirely, but replacing them with wholesome, all-natural ingredients that enhance the drinks.

- Incorporate as many skin-enhancing nutrients as possible into your drinks. Fruits, herbs, and roots that don't contain collagen are still great for your skin for other reasons—either they are packed with antioxidants that fight the toxins in your body, or are dense with nutrients that stimulate your body to produce more collagen.

Sweeteners and Milks

If the recipe calls for a certain sweetener or a milk, feel free to replace it with your favorite, or one that works the best for you:

SWEETENERS

- Lucuma powder (a Peruvian superfruit that goes perfect with milky bases)
- Agave nectar (goes perfect with juice bases)
- Honey (goes perfect with teas and juice bases)
- Bee pollen (goes perfect with teas)
- Stevia (goes perfect with juices and milk bases)
- Whole dates (goes perfect with milky shakes)
- Frozen banana (goes perfect with milky shakes)

MILKS

- Almond milk (goes with almost everything)
- Coconut milk (great with spices, such as turmeric)
- Cashew milk (a perfect coffee base)
- Oat milk
- Rice milk
- Pea milk (goes really well with matcha)
- Hemp milk

Caramel Rooibos Lucuma Latte

This lucuma latte is one of my personal favorites. Because it relies on lucuma powder, an all-natural, 0-calorie sweetener derived from a Peruvian fruit, for its sweet caramelly flavor instead of actual caramel, we get to forgo all the sugars that would spike your blood level afterward.

Makes 1 serving

½ cup hot water (too little water will make the rooibos taste too bitter)

1 rooibos tea bag

10 grams (about 1 tablespoon or scoop) collagen powder

1 tablespoon lucuma powder, plus more to garnish

1 cup almond milk

Pinch of ground cinnamon

TIP

If there are any clumps of powder, blend all the ingredients together, including the tea (this will actually give the latte a nice foamy layer at the top), or place the entire mixture in a saucepan and simmer together.

Brew the rooibos tea in the hot water.

Add the collagen powder and lucuma powder to the brewed tea.

Stir well.

Place the almond milk in a microwave-safe mug and heat in a microwave at a medium-high setting for 2 minutes.

Pour the heated almond milk into the rooibos tea mixture.

Sprinkle on more lucuma powder and cinnamon to taste.

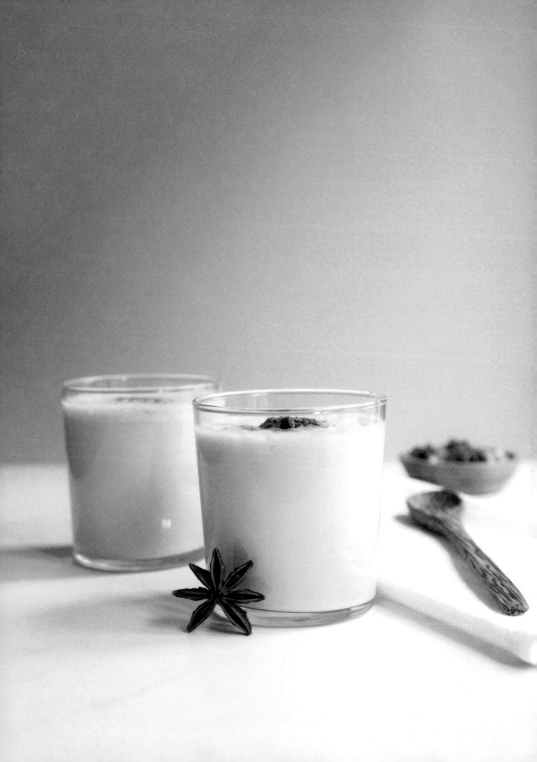

Matcha Tonic

My love for matcha runs deep: so deep that it's crowned itself as one of Crushed Tonic's flavors from day one. For those who aren't familiar with it, matcha is essentially green tea's better half (it's made by grinding high-quality, nutrient-rich green tea leaves into a fine powder). Matcha is ubiquitous in Korea—it is in our pastries and breads, desserts, and chocolates, and Koreans drink it almost as if it were water. And because the caffeine from the matcha is more of a soft lull, I usually don't feel the coffee crash that I often get after an espresso shot.

Makes 1 serving

1 teaspoon matcha powder

1 cup hot water plus ¼ cup lukewarm water for mixing

10 grams (about 1 tablespoon or scoop) collagen powder

TIP

If you don't have an electric milk frother, place the matcha powder into a water bottle or a canteen (even just 1 tablespoon of water is fine). Shake the bottle for 30 seconds. Add your collagen powder into the bottle using a funnel, then shake again. Add this mixture to a cup of hot water.

Pour the matcha powder into a glass containing about ¼ cup of lukewarm water.

Use an electric milk frother to whisk until all the matcha powder dissolves completely. Add the collagen powder, and whisk again.

Add the mixture to a mug of hot water. The less water, the deeper the matcha flavor profile will be; the more water added, the more it tastes like just any other green tea.

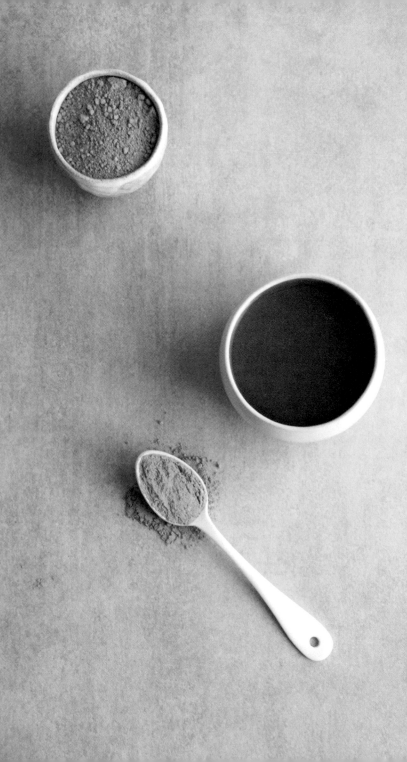

Iced Matcha Pea Milk Latte

Now that you know how to make a simple and soothing cup of simple matcha, I'll show you how to fall in love with it. Drinking matcha by itself is almost the same as drinking coffee black; it's doable, but definitely not as delicious as it could be.

This Earl Grey–infused matcha latte is a classy brunch favorite. By infusing the matcha into Earl Grey tea, you'll add hints of sophistication and elegance to the matcha, and the bergamot notes from the Earl Grey will enhance the whole experience. If Earl-Grey isn't your thing, feel free to get creative and combine matcha with fruity teas, such as raspberry teas (the process in mixing isn't too challenging—you just need to mix the matcha powder into already brewed tea).

Makes 1 serving

I make this collagen matcha latte almost every morning; it's become a ritual that I look forward to: not only does this latte achieve everything that a normal cup of matcha does, but because its base is nut milk, it's also incredibly satisfying and filling. And with more than 10 grams of protein (in addition to the 10 grams of protein from the collagen, pea milk is also a great source of plant-based protein) in it, I feel satiated and can go for hours without getting hungry. On days when I am rushing out the door, I know that I've found the perfect balance of filling and energizing by having this matcha latte.

¼ cup lukewarm water plus 1 mug of hot water for steeping

1 teaspoon matcha powder

10 grams (about 1 tablespoon or scoop) collagen powder

1 Earl Grey tea bag (optional)

1 cup pea milk, or your favorite nut milk

1 cup ice

Pour the lukewarm water into a reusable water bottle.

Add the matcha powder.

Shake until the matcha has completely dissolved.

Add the collagen powder to the water bottle.

Shake until both the collagen and matcha powder have completely dissolved.

If you'd like to add the Earl Grey tea, steep the tea bag in a mug of hot water for 2 minutes, then remove the tea bag. Add the tea to the water bottle and shake well.

Add the pea milk to the water bottle.

Shake well until the pea milk has infused with the matcha-infused elixir.

Pour the matcha latte into a glass.

Add the ice to the glass.

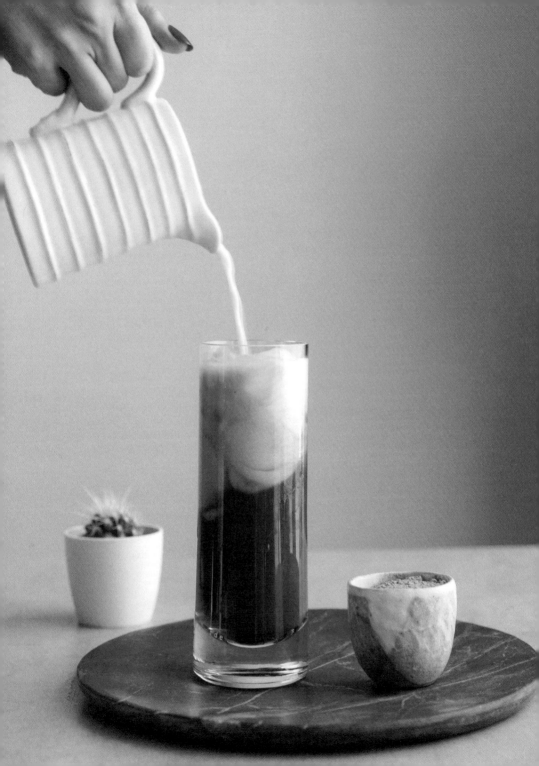

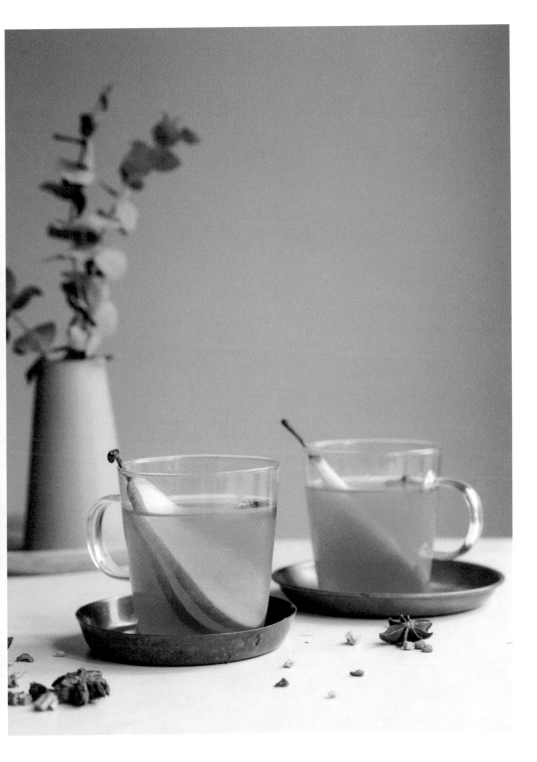

Mulled Apple and Pear Cider

Every winter, I make this mulled cider for my parents and grandparents and they go crazy for it. I like to add a splash of cider vinegar (one of my favorite things to drink daily as it helps me fight sugar cravings) to this recipe, and gift the mulled cider in recycled champagne bottles to hosts at holiday parties!

Makes 4 servings

8 apples, quartered

2 pears, quartered

6 dates

2 quarts filtered water

40 grams (about 4 tablespoons or 4 scoops) collagen powder

1 tablespoon ground cinnamon

1 tablespoon ground allspice

½ teaspoon grated nutmeg

Honey, or your favorite sweetener

Cider vinegar

Place the apples, pears, and dates in a 16-quart stockpot (it will overflow if it's not large enough) and add enough filtered water to cover the fruit by at least 3 inches.

Note that if you add too much water, the pot will overflow when it starts to boil—but if you don't add enough water, much of it will evaporate and you'll have to keep adding more water to the pot, which will dilute that nice apple cider taste.

Stir in the collagen powder, cinnamon, allspice, and nutmeg.

Bring to a boil and then continue to boil, uncovered, for 1 hour. Cover the pot, lower the heat to low, and simmer for 2 hours.

When the apples start to melt and disintegrate, you'll know that they are done.

Add honey to taste (the apples are already sweet enough, but honey helps bring it up a notch).

Place a cheesecloth or mesh net over a large bowl and strain the cider.

Add your desired number of drops of cider vinegar—it will add a tangy, faint kick to the cider, and pack in a ton of wellness!

Transfer the cider to a pitcher or champagne bottles.

Refrigerate until cold.

The acetic acid in cider vinegar has been shown to assist with weight loss due to its ability to inhibit lipogenesis (the formation of fat cells), lowering both waist size and body mass index (BMI).

55

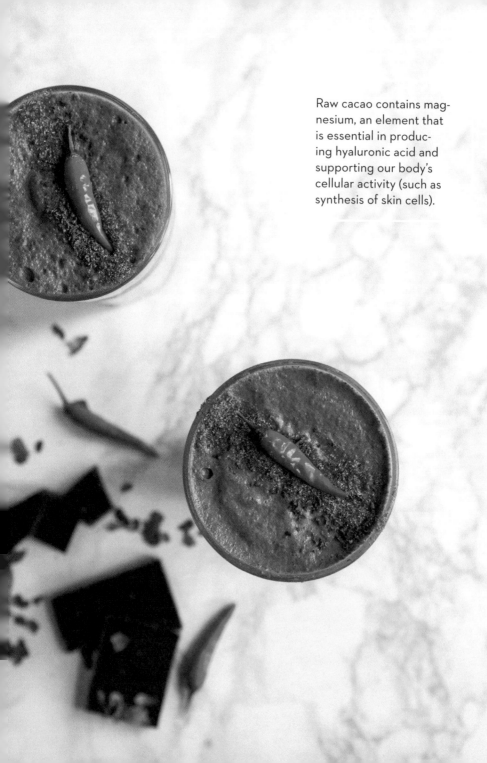

Raw cacao contains magnesium, an element that is essential in producing hyaluronic acid and supporting our body's cellular activity (such as synthesis of skin cells).

Chili Chocolate Chip Milk Shake

Who said all chocolate milk shakes had to be bad for you?

When I first moved to California and came across chocolate chip shakes, I was mind-blown. Not only was the shake creamy and chocolaty, it was blended with chocolate chips, for that satisfying, fun, and chocolaty crunch with every chocolaty sip (can you tell I love chocolate yet?!)—it was downright dreamy. But because it was so dense in sugar, I had to shy away from it—until I concocted this recipe.

This shake still allows for all the chocolate goodness: but because it is blended in harmony with antioxidants-loaded cacao powder and stevia-sweetened dark chocolate shavings—instead of the traditional sugar-packed chocolate chips—it comes with less than a fraction of that guilt.

I also like to add a pinch of cayenne pepper for an extra kick, but if you're not a fan of spices, feel free to leave it out, or add Himalayan sea salt instead.

Makes 1 serving

1 cup almond milk

10 grams (about 1 tablespoon or scoop) collagen powder

2 tablespoons raw cacao powder

1 to 3 drops pure vanilla extract

Pinch of ground cinnamon

Pinch of sea salt

Pinch of cayenne pepper

1 to 2 teaspoons lucuma powder, or your favorite sweetener

1 frozen banana

2 to 3 pieces stevia-sweetened dark chocolate

Place the almond milk, collagen powder, cacao powder, vanilla, cinnamon, sea salt, cayenne, lucuma powder, and frozen banana in a blender.

Wrap the dark chocolate in a paper towel. With the tips of a fork, break the chocolate into smaller pieces. Add the chocolate pieces to the blender. Blend well.

Honey Ginger Lemon Tea

Whenever I would tell my grandmother that I was feeling queasy, she would do two things: she would tie a thin string around my thumb and prick it at the top, and then she would proceed to spoon-feed me ladles of ginger tea. This ritual always made me feel better.

And it makes sense why: ginger is known to alleviate nausea and improve digestion, and to fight inflammation. As for the string around my thumb—I'm still not sure if that *actually* helped—but my grandmother swears by it. And of course, to soften the ginger taste, I recommend adding honey or your favorite sweetener to balance out the tangy taste of this magical root.

Makes 1 serving

10 grams (about 1 tablespoon or scoop) collagen powder

1 (2-inch) piece fresh organic ginger

1½ to 2 cups water

Juice of 2 lemons

1 to 2 tablespoons yuzu honey, or your favorite sweetener

Peel and slice the ginger.

Boil the ginger in the water for at least 10 minutes.

Add the lemon juice. Remove from the heat and add the yuzu honey to taste.

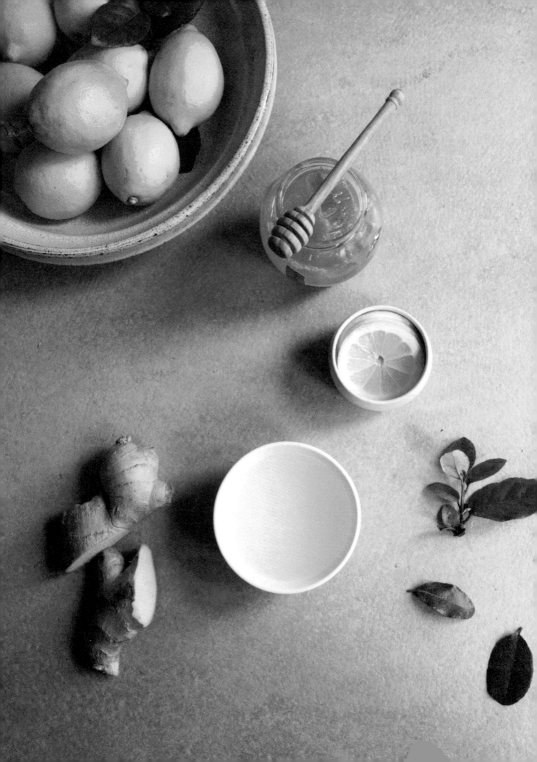

Avocados are packed with folate and potassium, while dark leafy greens, such as kale and spinach, are great for your eyes and for increasing hyaluronic acid levels, as they are high in magnesium.

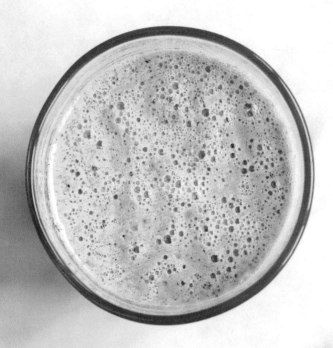

Avocado Banana Greens Smoothie

Ah, millennials and our obsession with avocados. And it doesn't stop at avo toasts. But because I try to keep a gluten-free diet for the most part, I actually prefer this filling shake over toast—especially because I can make this smoothie with kale, spinach, and other not-as-delicious superfoods that I can't taste amid the avocado bliss. This shake is perfect as a breakfast-to-go, an afternoon pick-me-up, or a booster right before your workout class.

Makes 1 serving

10 grams (about 1 tablespoon or scoop) collagen powder

1 avocado, peeled and pitted

1 teaspoon olive oil

Handful of kale

Handful of spinach

1 frozen banana

1 cup almond milk, or your favorite milk

Combine the collagen powder, avocado, olive oil, kale, spinach, frozen banana, and almond milk in a blender and blend.

TIP

You can turn this into avocado banana ice cream—just start off with only about ¼ cup of almond milk, and add ice. Blitz and blitz in a blender until you have a consistency similar to that of ice cream. Add a pinch of salt for a more savory flavor.

Chocolate Horchata

Here's a wellness spin on horchata, an indulgent Mexican drink made from soaked rice, cream, and sugar that I used to drink regularly growing up in California. Instead of the sugar bomb of the original, I turned to rice milk with vanilla extract. I like to add ample amounts of cinnamon, too, as it's great for heart health!

Makes 1 serving

2 to 3 pieces stevia-sweetened dark chocolate

1 cup rice milk

10 grams (about 1 tablespoon or scoop) collagen powder

1 teaspoon ground cinnamon

1 to 3 drops pure vanilla extract

2 teaspoons lucuma powder, or your favorite sweetener

Wrap the dark chocolate in a paper towel. With the tips of a fork, break the chocolate into smaller pieces.

Blend all the ingredients together and sweeten to taste.

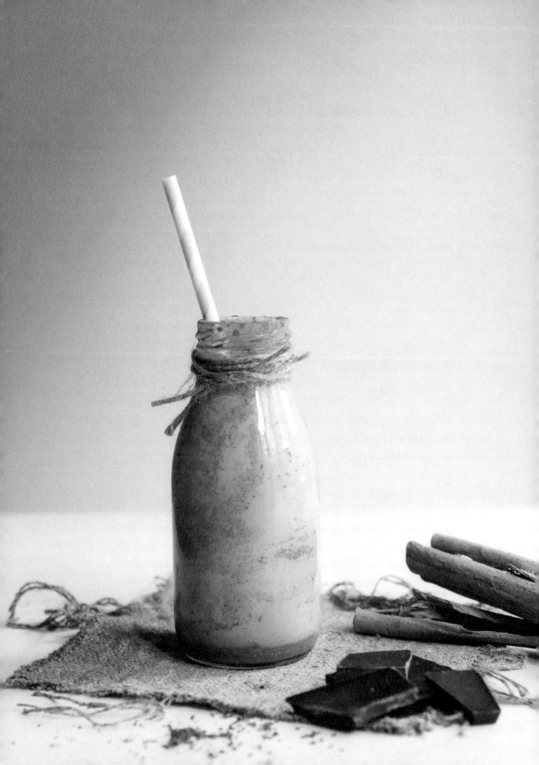

Açai Crunch Smoothie

I fell in love with açai bowls in Puerto Rico—so much so that I had it every meal during a visit there. I'm still just as obsessed: not only is it tropical and sweet, the dollop of almond butter fills you up in the hottest of summers (but not bloated enough to take you off the beach). This recipe has turned the cult favorite, the açai bowl, into a wellness smoothie!

Makes 1 serving

½ beet (optional)

2 frozen bananas, divided

1 cup frozen raspberries

1 tablespoon water

2 tablespoons almond butter

1 cup toasted granola

10 grams (about 1 tablespoon or scoop) collagen powder

1 cup açai puree

1 cup almond milk or your favorite milk, plus more for blending

Coconut flakes, for garnish

Blueberries, for garnish

Place the beet, one frozen banana, frozen berries, and water in a blender and blend together.

Pour the mixture into a glass.

Layer the almond butter on top of the puree.

Layer the granola on top.

Combine the collagen, açai puree, almond milk, and remaining frozen banana in a blender. Add more almond milk as you blend, but slowly, to achieve the consistency you want.

Pour on top of the other layered ingredients.

Sprinkle with coconut flakes and fresh blueberries before serving.

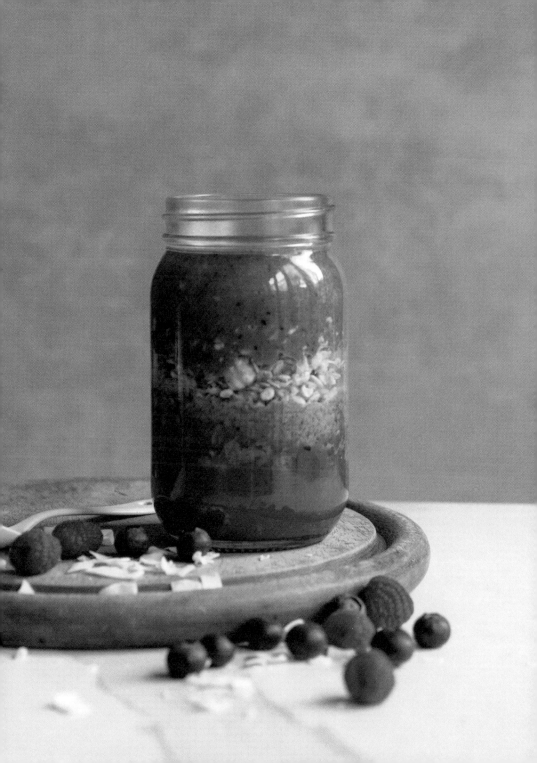

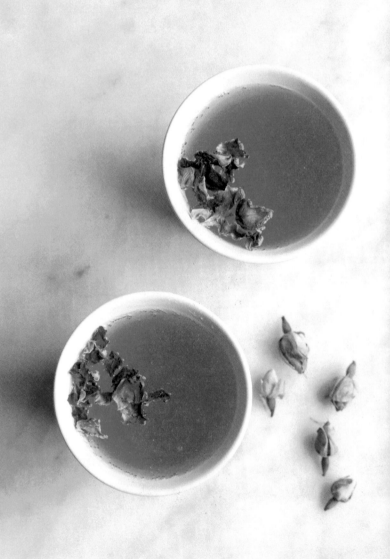

Rose Water Tonic

Rose water has a lot of benefits: it's great for both ingestible and topical usage. So, not only do I add a splash of rose water to everything I drink, especially all of my cocktails, I like to spritz it on topically whenever I wake up to freshen up my skin, before applying any moisturizer. It instantly hydrates your skin and gives you that instant refreshed look and feel, on top of leaving this sweet and clean scent. Fun fact—apparently it was one of Cleopatra's (yes, Cleopatra from Egyptian ancient times) favorite skincare rituals!

Makes 1 serving

¼ cup dried organic food-grade rose petals, or ½ cup fresh

1½ cups filtered water

10 grams (about 1 tablespoon or scoop) of collagen powder

One 12-ounce can seltzer water per serving

> Rose water contains quercetin and kaempferol, which may improve sore throat symptoms and skin irritation by protecting fibroblast cells from oxidative damage.

Place the rose petals in a small, lidded saucepan and add the filtered water.

Cover and bring to a boil.

Lower the heat to the lowest setting that still allows the water to simmer.

Simmer for 5 minutes.

Remove from the heat, leave the lid on, and let cool completely.

Place a cheesecloth over a medium bowl. Strain the mixture through the cheesecloth.

To prepare each drink, mix the collagen with 1 tablespoon of rose water in a glass until it's dissolved. Top off with the seltzer.

Store the remaining rose water in the refrigerator for up to one week.

Tropical Smoothie with Ginger Boost

This smoothie is a perfect mixture of the Caribbean Islands and the Far East: on top of the sweet mango flavor, the ginger gives it a spicy kick. In addition to its diverse flavor makeup, this smoothie has many anti-aging and immunity-boosting benefits, as mango, passion fruit, coconut, and ginger all contain incredible antioxidants, flavonoids, and vitamins.

Makes 1 serving

2 ripe passion fruits

10 grams (about 1 tablespoon or scoop) of collagen powder

1 frozen banana

½ cup mango chunks

½ cup red apple chunks

One 1-inch piece fresh ginger

½ cup coconut milk

¼ cup organic orange juice

2 tablespoons coconut milk yogurt

Ice cubes (optional)

Cut each passion fruit in half and scoop out the seeds to save for later (to top the smoothie). The flesh will be used in the smoothie.

Place the passion fruit, collagen powder, frozen banana, mango, apple, ginger, coconut milk, orange juice, and yogurt in a blender.

Blend, adding ice to bring the mixture to your desired consistency.

Top with the reserved passion fruit seeds.

Passion fruits are dense in fiber—one fruit provides the human body with approximately 98 percent of our daily fiber requirement—while mangos are a great source of phytochemicals, such as resveratrol and quercetin, which can help with weight loss and improve digestion.

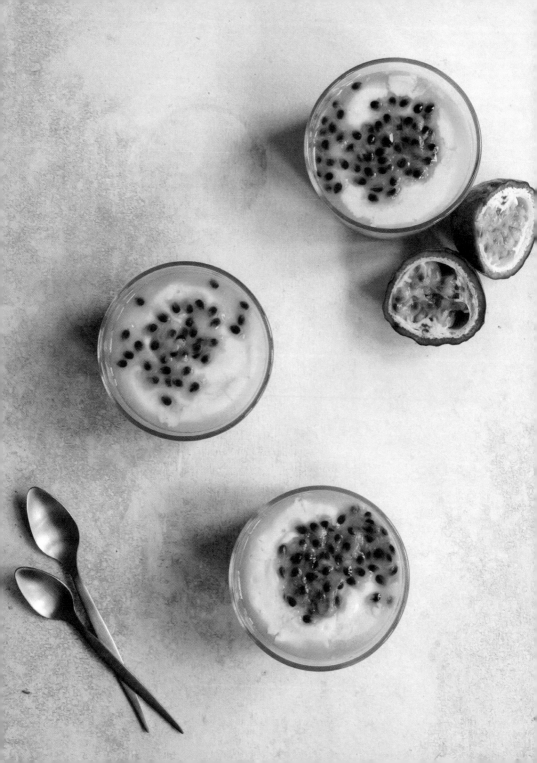

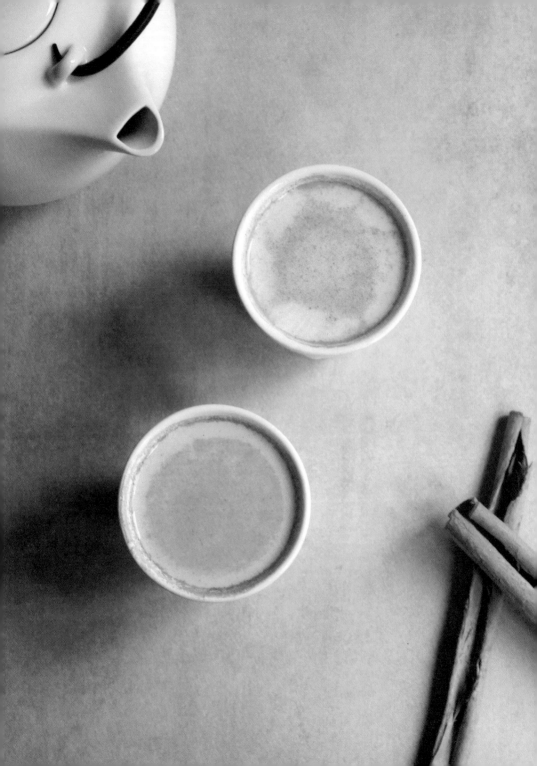

Golden Milk Turmeric Latte

Whenever I'm coming down with something, I like to drink this twice a day. And it's like magic—within 48 hours, I feel so much better again. Fun fact? The turmeric in this magic concoction has been used by Ayurvedic healers for thousands of years!

Makes 1 serving

1 cup unsweetened almond milk or pea milk

½ cup water

10 grams (about 1 tablespoon or scoop) collagen powder

½ teaspoon ground turmeric

Pinch of ground ginger

Pinch of ground cinnamon

Freshly ground black pepper

1 teaspoon grated fresh ginger

Combine the almond milk, water, collagen powder, turmeric, ground ginger, and cinnamon in a saucepan.

Simmer over medium heat until all the powder has dissolved.

Sprinkle the black pepper and grated ginger on top to serve.

If you are unfamiliar with the powers of turmeric, this ancient root is a cousin of ginger that is said to boost our immune system's defense mechanisms, enhance metabolism, increase our white blood cell count, aiding against bacteria and viruses, and support in our liver detoxification process. It is also reported to increase our body's collagen synthesis, in addition to helping aid cell regeneration (which allows for faster wound healing).

Homemade Chocolate Almond Milk

It's actually very simple to make homemade almond milk—and because I know exactly what's going inside, I don't feel guilty at all when I overindulge. (Yes, it's possible—I've downed a whole pitcher of this stuff in one sitting.)

Makes 2 servings

1 cup almonds

2 cups filtered water, plus more for soaking

1 large pitted date

2 tablespoons raw cacao powder

1 teaspoon ground cinnamon

Sea salt

Agave nectar, or your favorite sweetener

Place the almonds in a bowl or jar and cover with filtered water. Cover and soak overnight.

Drain and rinse the almonds, discarding the soaking liquid.

Transfer the almonds to a blender and add the 2 cups of filtered water, the date, the cacao powder, cinnamon, and sea salt. Blend until smooth.

Place a cheesecloth over a bowl and strain the almond mixture to separate the liquid from the pulp. Discard the pulp.

Sweeten the chocolate almond milk with agave to taste. Use within 24 hours.

TIP

If you can't finish this within 24 hours, do what I love to do: freeze the milk in an ice cube tray and snack on them for dessert.

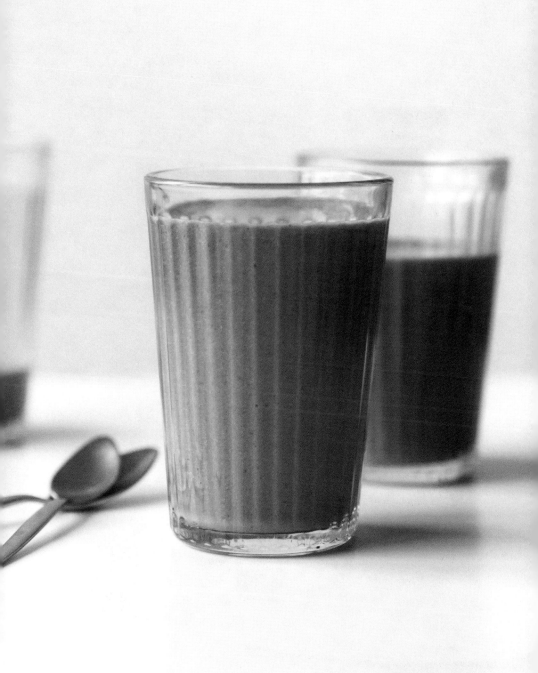

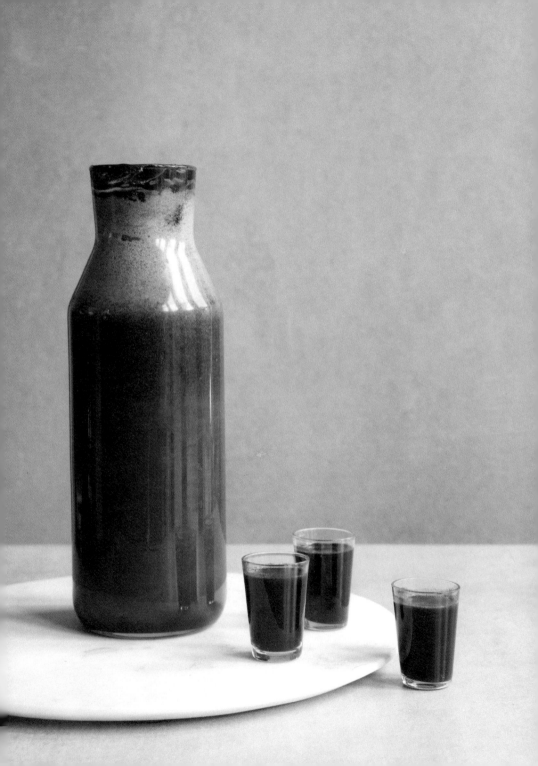

Spirulina Chlorophyll Tonic

Spirulina is a king of superfoods. It is a complete protein that is rich in vitamin C, A, magnesium, iron, calcium, AND chlorophyll! So, as you can imagine, a shot of this ticks off many boxes of one's wellness routine.

Makes 1 serving

10 grams (about 1 tablespoon or scoop) collagen powder

2 teaspoons spirulina powder

1 cup filtered water

Place all the ingredients in a blender.

Blend.

Peppermint Matcha Latte

I love anything and everything peppermint. But who am I kidding, I love mint really anytime of the year. This creamy, minty matcha latte is refreshing and energizing—perfect as dessert after a heavy meal.

Makes 1 serving

1 cup almond milk

½ cup water

10 grams (about 1 tablespoon or scoop) collagen powder

2 teaspoons matcha powder

¼ teaspoon peppermint extract

Agave nectar, or your favorite sweetener

Combine the almond milk, water, collagen powder, matcha powder, peppermint extract, and agave in a saucepan.

Simmer over medium heat until all the powder has dissolved.

Try not to let the matcha boil—it can lose its antioxidants and take on a bitter taste.

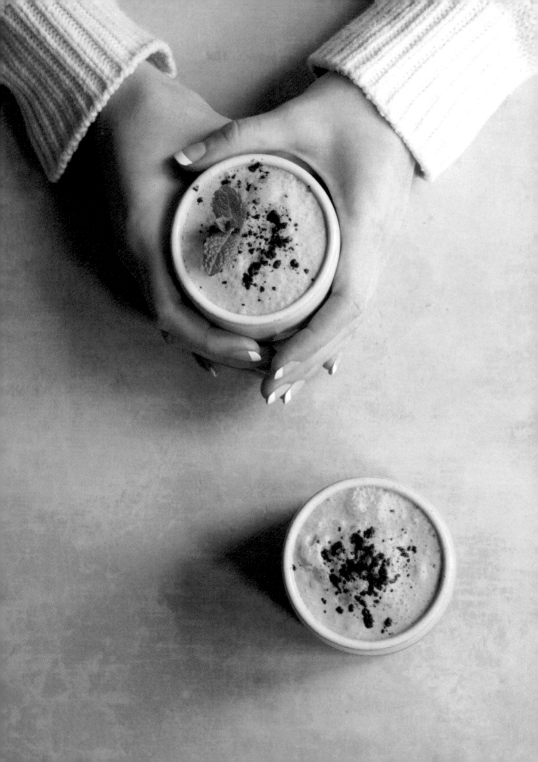

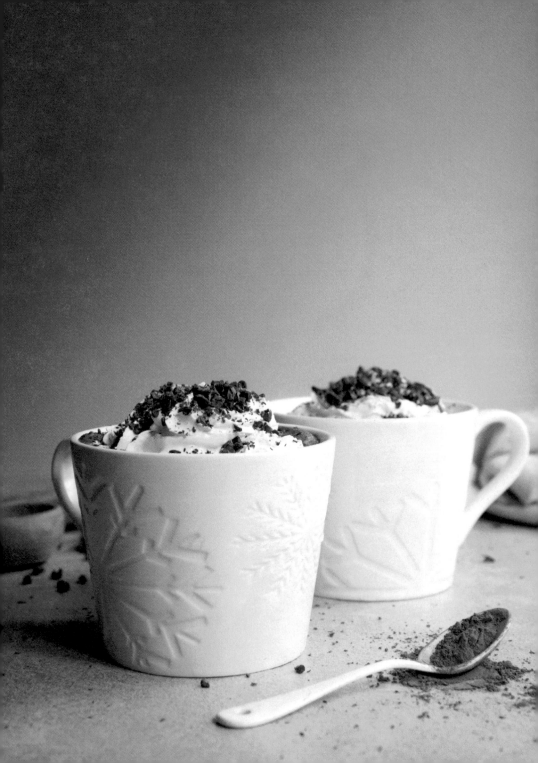

Hot Cacao + Mushroom Ceremony Elixir

This is an adult version of hot cocoa, my favorite childhood drink. Despite retaining the chocolaty goodness, there is zero refined sugar added to it, and it is enhanced in function and benefits with medicinal mushrooms. The thought of drinking mushrooms may seem foreign to some; I definitely felt that when I was first introduced to it. But because my grandmother loved mushrooms, I learned to appreciate and now love it.

After a long day, I like to cradle a huge mug of this elixir, sit in front of my favorite candle, ruminate on the day, and meditate. This ritual keeps me centered; and with the fragrance of the cacao, it's truly a one-of-a-kind elixir.

Makes 1 serving

1 cup boiling water

10 grams (about 1 tablespoon or scoop) collagen powder

2 to 3 tablespoons raw cacao powder

1 teaspoon Cordyceps powder

1 to 2 teaspoons coconut oil (optional)

1 teaspoon lucuma powder (optional)

1 cup unsweetened almond milk

Pinch of sea salt

Coconut Whipped Cream (recipe follows) or store-bought non-dairy whipped cream

In a saucepan, combine the boiling water, collagen powder, cacao powder, Cordyceps powder, and the oil and lucuma powder, if using, and stir well.

Add the almond milk, sprinkle with a pinch of sea salt, and stir again.

Coconut Whipped Cream

If you're in the mood for something sweet, add more cacao and lucuma powder to taste, and top off with coconut whipped cream (which no hot chocolate is complete without!).

Makes 2 cups

One 14-ounce can coconut milk

1 teaspoon pure vanilla extract

Stevia, or your favorite sweetener

Refrigerate the can of coconut milk overnight.

Scoop the coconut cream solids into a cold mixing bowl.

Beat the coconut cream with an electric mixer on medium speed for 10 minutes.

Add the vanilla and your favorite sweetener to the bowl. Beat for 1 more minute.

Medicinal mushrooms, such as Cordyceps, help support your liver and kidneys, and are known to help keep your cortisol levels low (which prevents the breakdown of your body's own collagen), and contain proteoglycan, a collagen production supporter. Cordyceps also contain glutathione, which is known to help reduce inflammation.

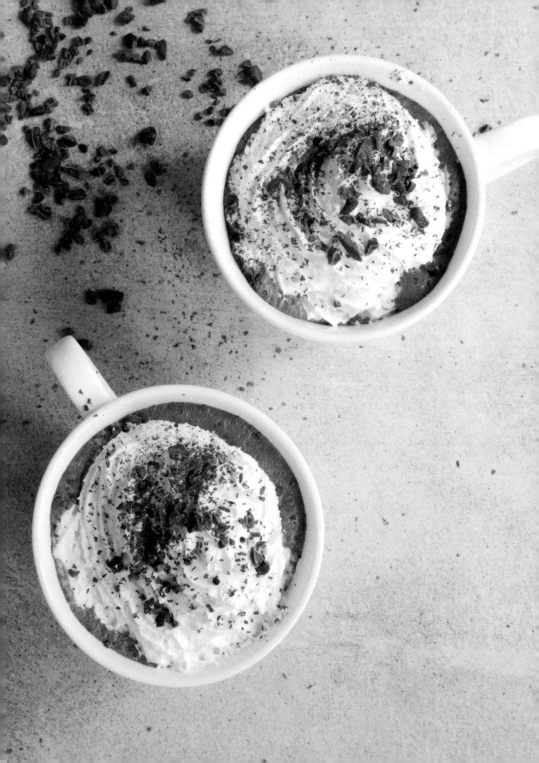

Persimmon Iced Latte

Frozen, thawed, ripened persimmons are an incredibly delicious dessert. My *emo* (my aunt) likes to freeze a dozen ripe persimmons, and then move them to the fridge overnight so that they thaw, and takes one out before we start having dinner so we can have one as dessert, as they turn into a cool, sorbet/ ice cream–like texture that melts in your mouth.

Makes 1 serving

10 grams (about 1 tablespoon or scoop) collagen powder

1 frozen, then thawed, Korean persimmon (*hachiya*)

½ cup water

1 cup coconut milk, or your favorite milk

Place all the ingredients in a blender and blend.

> **TIP**
>
> Korean persimmons (*hachiya*) are squishy and fleshy, not hard. You can find them in Korean markets or some specialty food stores. The recipe can be made with other types of persimmons, but make sure they are very ripe.

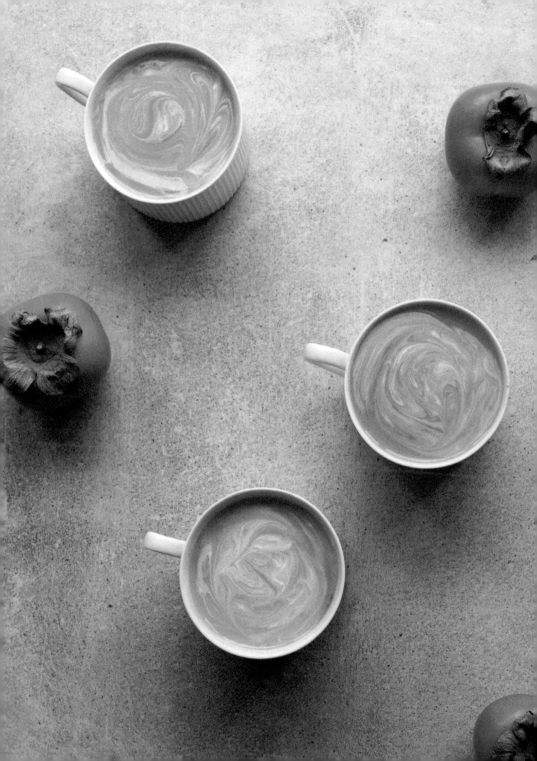

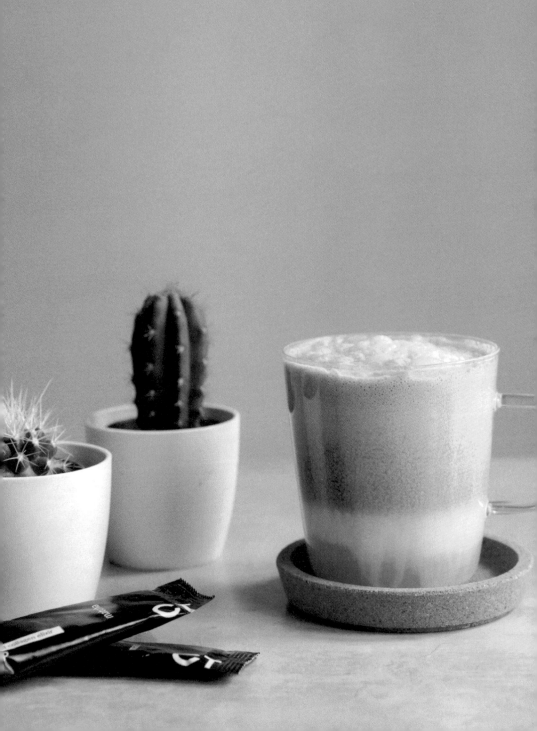

Pandan Maca Latte

My most life-changing trip was to Bali, Indonesia. The beaches, the temples, the people—and of course, the food! My favorite culinary discovery was pandan—these sweet, tropical, vanilla-y leaves that many Indonesians boil and add to enhance their teas.

Makes 1 serving

10 cups boiling water

6 pieces of pandan leaves

10 grams (about 1 tablespoon or scoop) collagen powder

1 teaspoon maca powder

1 tablespoon of your favorite sweetener

1 cup of your favorite milk

> Pandan leaves are known to help relieve headaches and lower stress levels, while maca has been used for centuries to improve mood and energy.

Add the pandan leaves to the boiling water.

Once you see that the pandan leaves have been cooked thoroughly and there is a yellowish tint to the boiling water, drain the pandan water into a bowl.

Combine 1 cup of the pandan water and the collagen, maca, and your favorite sweetener in a saucepan. Discard the remaining pandan water. Add your favorite milk and bring to a simmer, then serve.

Overnight Cold Brew

For me, coffee is sacred, which is why I'd never liked adding collagen to it. But now that I've found the collagen powder that works for me, I am able to add it to coffee without being turned off by it. So here's a coffee connoisseur-approved recipe, to be prepped before a schedule-packed day. Combined with the 10 grams of protein and oat milk, it is filling and delicious, and will fuel you for the entire morning!

Makes 6 servings

1 cup coffee beans (more for a darker roast)

About 8 cups filtered water, divided

10 grams (about 1 tablespoon or scoop) collagen powder

Milk of your choice

> **TIP**
>
> Some of my favorite treats growing up were Vietnamese and Thai iced coffees.

Grind the coffee beans to the consistency of bread crumbs. Transfer to a large pitcher.

Pour 7 cups of the filtered water into the pitcher. Stir well and steep for 18 to 24 hours in the fridge.

The next day, cover a large bowl with cheesecloth and strain the mixture into the bowl. Repeat two or three times, until all the residue is gone and you are left with a liquid cold brew concentrate.

To serve, dissolve the collagen in a tablespoon of water in a glass. Add water and coffee concentrate, two parts water to one part coffee. Stir in milk of your choice and serve over ice.

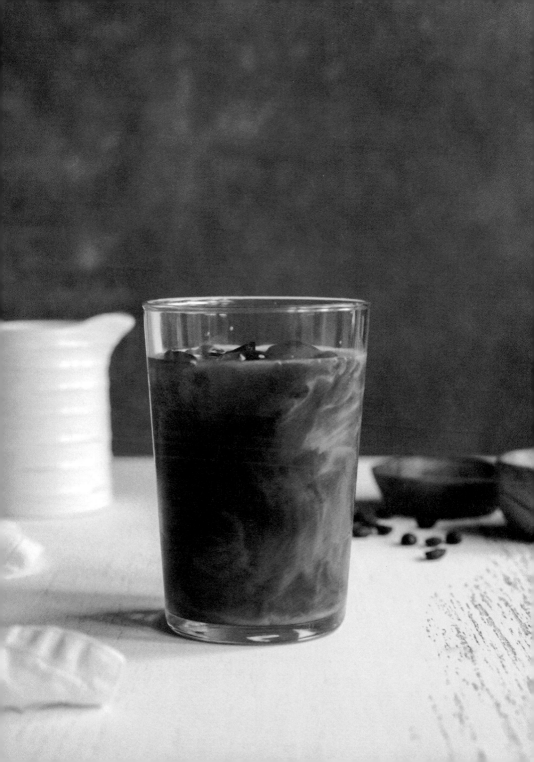

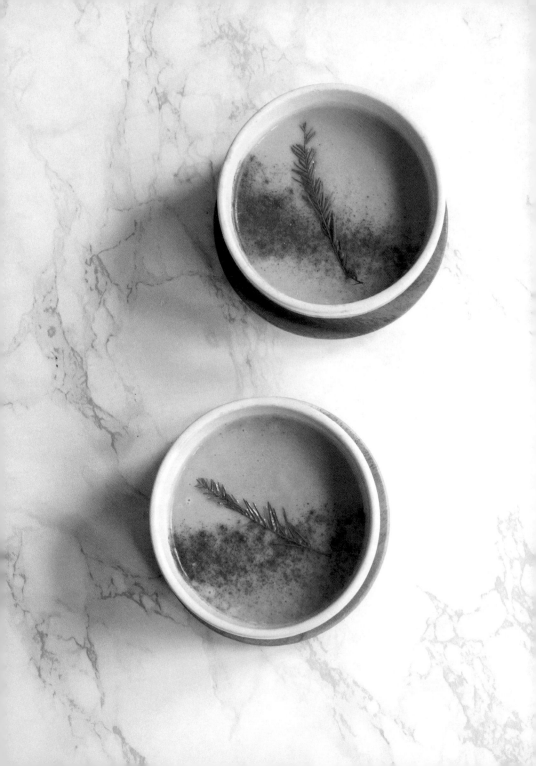

Sweet Potato Latte

This fall, instead of the pumpkin spice latte, reach for a creamy sweet potato latte instead. These healthful sweet potato lattes are loved so much in Korea that you can find them at almost every coffee chain (even the Korean Starbucks) and juice cafés.

Makes 1 serving

1 small sweet potato

10 grams (about 1 tablespoon or scoop) of collagen powder

1¼ cups unsweetened almond milk

Pinch of ground cinnamon (optional)

Sweet potatoes are an excellent source of vitamin A and are great for your skin, from head to toe, and can keep you feeling full and satiated for hours.

Steam the sweet potato until it is fully cooked and soft, 20 to 25 minutes.

Once the sweet potato is ready, put the steamed sweet potato flesh and the collagen powder and almond milk into a blender. Add the cinnamon, if using. Blend until the mixture is perfectly homogenized.

Vanilla Lemon Latte

This vanilla latte is a favorite of my family and friends: it's bittersweet, relaxing, and sophisticated. I love it with a spritz of lemon!

Makes 1 serving

1 cup almond milk

¼ teaspoon pure vanilla extract

2 dates

10 grams (about 1 tablespoon or scoop) collagen powder

Honey, or your favorite sweetener

Lemon wedge

> Drinking lemon is known to aid with digestion, as it contains limonene, compounds that can assist with weight loss and fighting inflammation!

Microwave the almond milk on medium power for 2 minutes.

Combine the hot almond milk, vanilla extract, dates, and collagen powder in a blender. Blend on high speed until smooth and creamy.

Add honey to taste.

Spritz with lemon juice before serving and drink immediately.

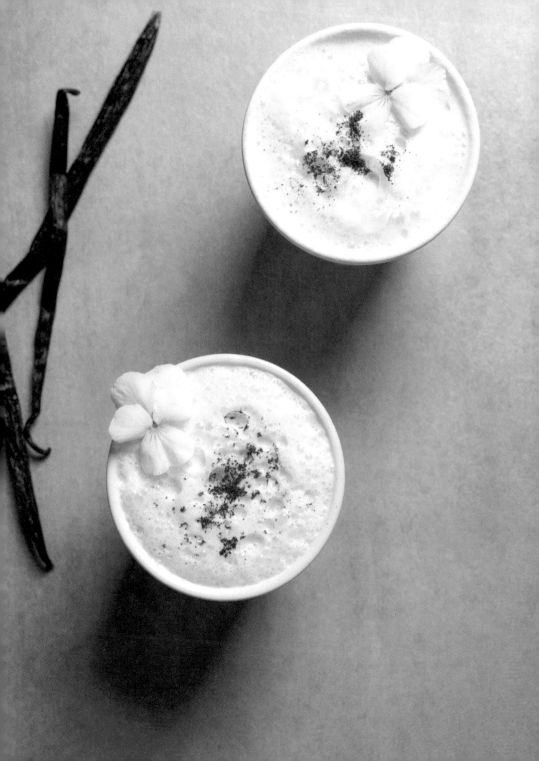

Upside-Down Chocolate-Covered Raspberry Smoothie

This playful take on chocolate-covered berries is a satisfying, low-sugar treat. You can make the chocolate pudding ahead of time and serve it by itself, or make yourself an upside-down smoothie by layering the chocolate on the bottom, then adding the raspberry mixture, and sprinkling more shaved chocolate and freeze-dried raspberries on top. The creamy chocolate, the icy fruit, and the crispy toppings are a delicious trio of texture and flavors.

Makes 2 servings

CHOCOLATE PUDDING

2½ cups coconut milk

½ cup chia seeds

6 tablespoons raw cacao powder

1 tablespoon lucuma powder

½ teaspoon pure vanilla extract

Pinch of salt

RASPBERRY SMOOTHIE

20 grams (about 2 tablespoons or scoops) collagen powder

1 frozen banana

2 cups frozen raspberries

1 cup almond milk

TO SERVE

1 to 2 pieces stevia-sweetened dark chocolate shavings

1 teaspoon freeze-dried fruit, crushed (I used a mix of raspberries and apples)

> Raspberries are packed with ellagic acid, antioxidants that can help fight signs of aging, such as wrinkles.

TO MAKE THE CHOCOLATE PUDDING

Combine all the pudding ingredients in a blender.

Let the pudding sit on the counter or in the refrigerator for at least 10 to 15 minutes. It can be refrigerated up to 24 hours.

TO MAKE THE RASPBERRY SMOOTHIE

Place the collagen powder, frozen banana, raspberries, and almond milk in a blender and blend well.

Serve immediately.

TO SERVE

Place a cup of pudding in a wide-bottomed glass. Layer on half of the smoothie mixture, and sprinkle with toppings. Serve immediately.

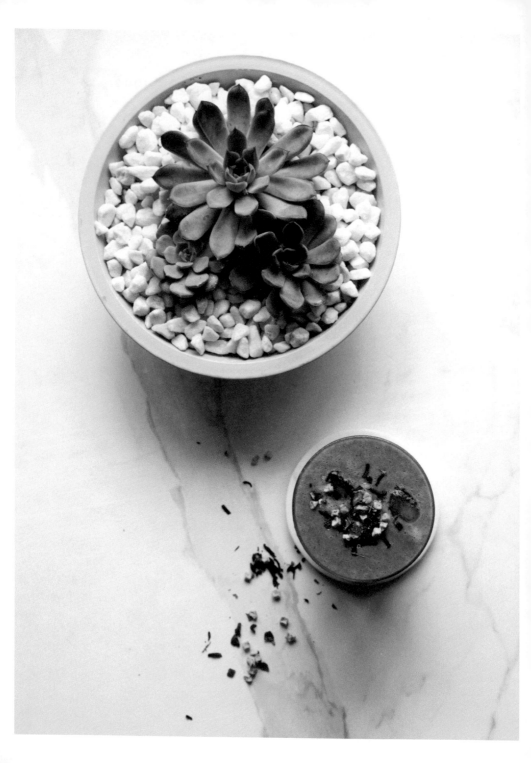

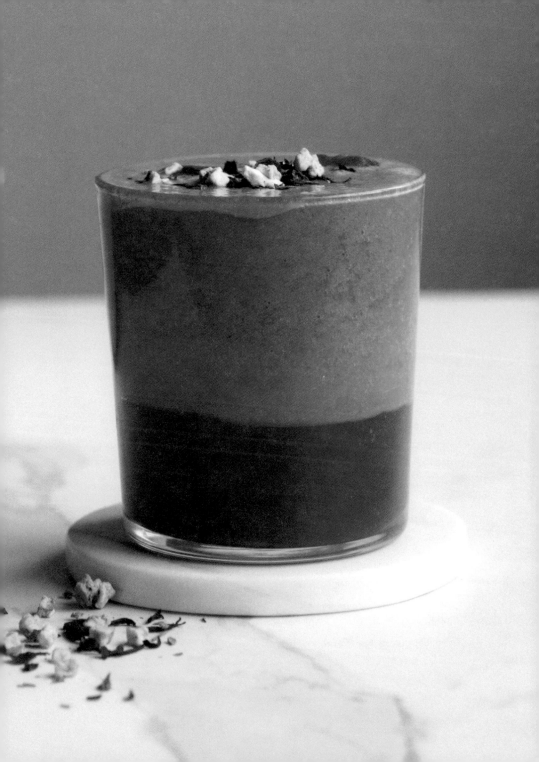

Mango Turmeric Lassi

This is a wellness-spin on one of the world's most treasured drinks—the mango lassi. Mango lassi—sweet, creamy, and refreshing—is, of course, as amazing as it comes on its own, and doesn't necessarily need any improvements. But I actually love it even more when I add a pinch of turmeric to it—it gives it a wholesome, savory twist.

Makes 1 serving

10 grams (about 1 tablespoon or scoop) collagen powder

1 tablespoon filtered water

1 cup chopped mango

½ cup Greek yogurt

½ cup coconut water

½ cup coconut milk, plus more if desired

½ cup organic orange juice (optional)

4 teaspoons honey, or your favorite sweetener

Ice

Pinch of ground turmeric

Pinch of ground cardamom (optional)

Pinch of grated nutmeg (optional)

Combine the collagen with the filtered water in a blender.

Add the mango, yogurt, coconut water, coconut milk, orange juice, honey, turmeric, cardamom, and nutmeg, if using, and blend for 2 minutes.

Add ice and more coconut milk to achieve your desired consistency.

To serve, sprinkle with a tiny pinch of ground cardamom, nutmeg, and turmeric, if desired.

> Turmeric goes well with citrusy and tropical fruits and juices—apple juice, orange juice, grapefruit juice, lemonade, and of course, mango juice!

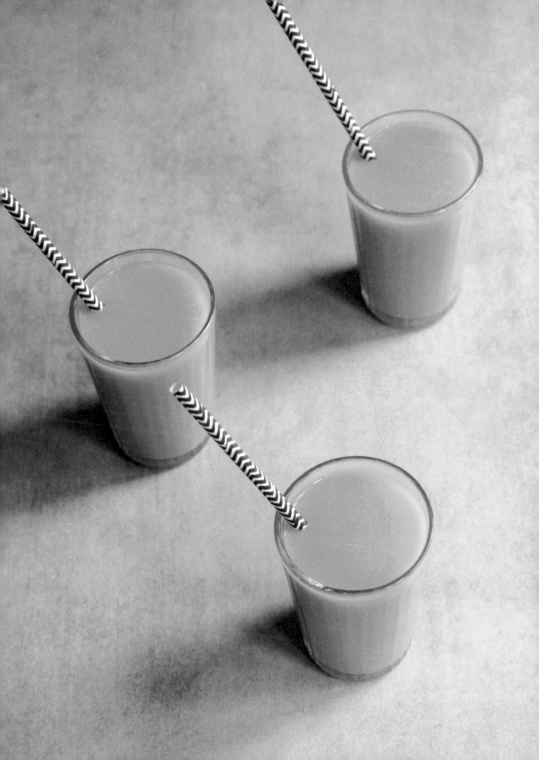

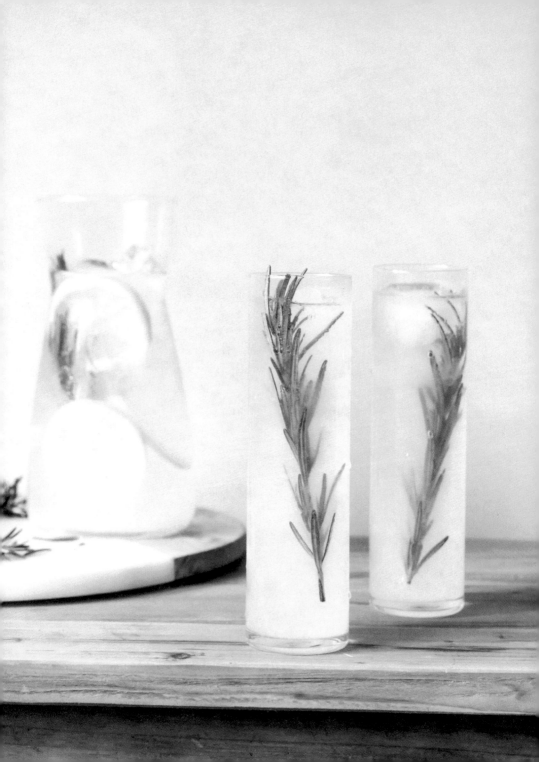

Rosemary Lemonade

A lemonade for the "grown-ups." Our childhood favorite, combined with an herbal, woody note of rosemary—perfect for a barbecue with friends and family in the summer!

Makes 2 servings

20 grams (about 2 tablespoons or scoops) collagen powder

1 to 2 cup filtered water

4 lemons

1 sprig of rosemary

Agave nectar

Rosemary is known to improve memory and may even help prevent the spread of skin cancer.

Mix the collagen into the filtered water in a pitcher.

Squeeze the lemons into the pitcher.

Drop in the rosemary. Let it steep in the lemonade for 30 minutes or more before serving.

Sweeten with agave nectar, as desired.

Pineapple and Kiwi Coconut Slushie

This pineapple kiwi slushie is rejuvenating and refreshing—not to mention fun and a true ice-breaker at potlucks!

Makes 1 serving

GREEN SLUSHIE

2 cups of your favorite milk

2 tablespoons wheatgrass powder

20 grams (about 2 tablespoons or scoops) collagen powder

2 handfuls of your favorite greens: kale and spinach

2 ripe kiwi fruits, peeled

1 frozen banana

TO MAKE THE GREEN SLUSHIE

Place ingredients in the blender in the order they appear, and blend well. Pour into two large glasses or jars. Rinse the blender and make the pineapple mixture.

PINEAPPLE SLUSHIE

½ cup coconut water

½ cup coconut milk

1 pineapple core, chopped

1 cup ice (more if needed)

TO MAKE THE PINEAPPLE SLUSHIE

Place ingredients in blender in the order they appear and blend until smooth. This should be light and fluffy, so add more ice if needed. Layer the pineapple mixture on top of the kiwi mixture and serve.

Kiwis are a great source of antioxidants, such as lutein, and eating them may lower blood pressure and improve digestion.

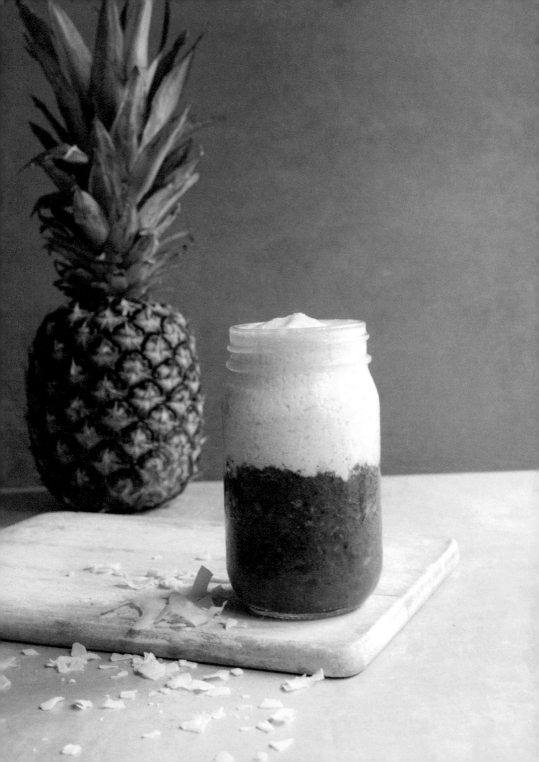

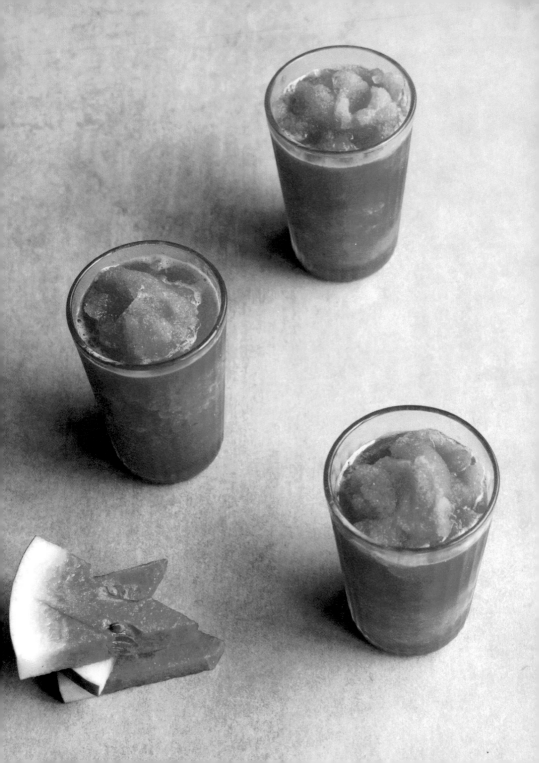

Watermelon Cucumber Slushie

In Korea, watermelon and cucumbers are iconic skincare foods, both eaten and applied directly to skin: whenever I would get sunburnt, my grandmother would use thin slices of chilled watermelon and cucumbers to soothe my inflamed skin. But who am I kidding; I ate watermelon like it was candy—be it beneficial or not, I still will often finish off an entire melon in one sitting!

Makes 2 servings

2½ pounds watermelon

1/4 cucumber

20 grams (about 2 tablespoons or scoops) collagen powder

1 cup ice

1 to 3 teaspoons agave nectar or honey, or sweetener of your choice

Scoop out the watermelon flesh, removing as many seeds as possible.

Slice the cucumber as thinly as possible.

Place the melon, cucumber, collagen powder, ice, and agave in a blender and blend together.

Made mostly of water, watermelons are amazing in keeping you feel hydrated and energized. In addition, because watermelon is packed with potassium, lycopene, vitamins A, B6, and C, not only are they great for your eyes and immunity, they are terrific for your skin: from the inside out.

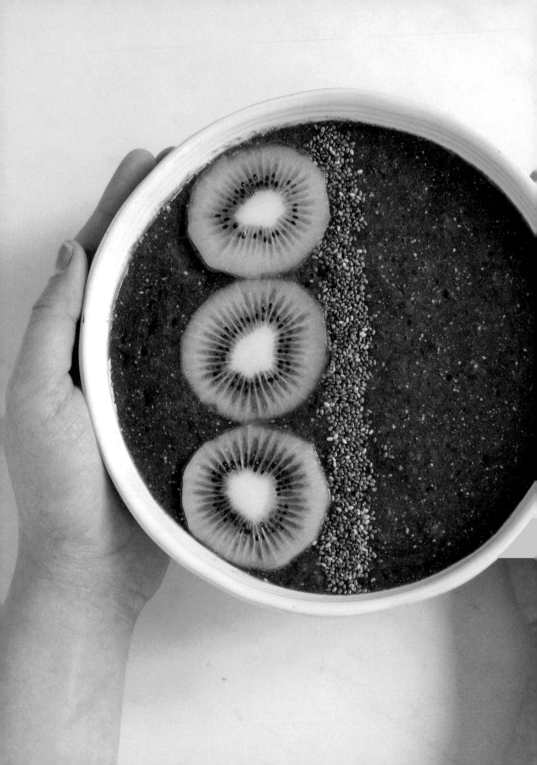

Smoothie Bowls

Coconut Vanilla Fig Smoothie Bowl

This may be my favorite dessert of all. It's supereasy to make, scrumptious, filling, tastes like ice cream, *and* is low in calories—whoever thought these words could all be in the same sentence?

Makes 1 serving

10 grams (about 1 tablespoon or scoop) collagen

1 tablespoon water

1 frozen banana

1 cup of your favorite milk

1 to 2 cups ice

1 tablespoon coconut milk

1 fig, sliced

1 tablespoon goji berries

Stir the collagen into 1 tablespoon of the water.

Stir well and then transfer the mixture to a blender.

Add the frozen banana, milk, ice, and coconut milk to the blender.

Blitz, pausing every 2 seconds to ensure that the consistency is more like ice cream than a smoothie.

Scoop out with a big serving spoon.

Add sliced fig and goji berries before serving.

I love adding goji berries to smoothie bowls for that exotic and chewy texture. But not only are they fun to chew, goji berries are great for you: they are packed with antiaging properties and are also known to help reduce fatigue and stress.

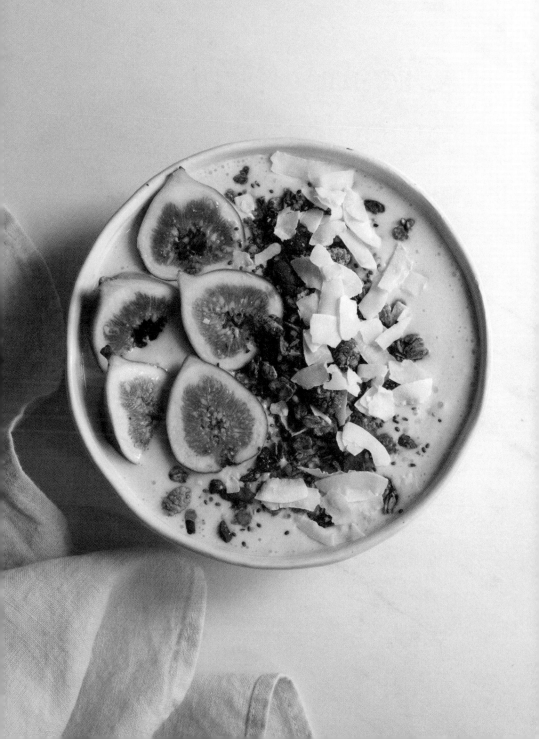

Creamy Orange Smoothie

This smoothie bowl is a re-creation of the orange Creamsicle pop, my childhood favorite—creamy with a perfect hint of citrus.

Makes 1 serving

10 grams (about 1 tablespoon or scoop) collagen powder

1 tablespoon water

1 to 3 drops pure vanilla extract

1 frozen banana

1 cup of your favorite milk

1 to 2 cups ice

1 peeled orange or ½ cup fresh juice

Stir the collagen into 1 tablespoon of the water. Stir well and then transfer the mixture to a blender.

Add the rest of the ingredients and blend well.

Oranges are often recommended to be consumed with collagen as they contain vitamin C, which our body relies on to produce collagen.

Fun fact: Collagen and the extracellular matrix of the skin cannot be synthesized unless vitamin C is found in the body in adequate amounts!

Vitamin C also helps amino acids convert to collagen. As an antioxidant, vitamin C is water-soluble and reduces levels of free radicals linked with aging of the skin. Vitamin C also increases moisture of the skin through increases in collagen synthesis.

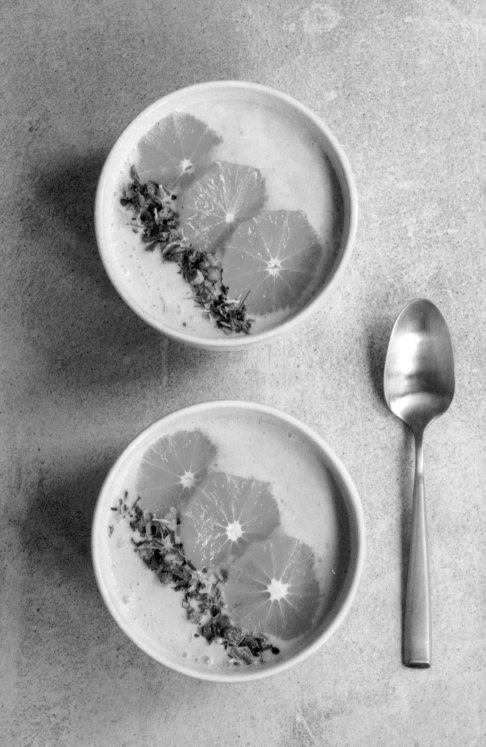

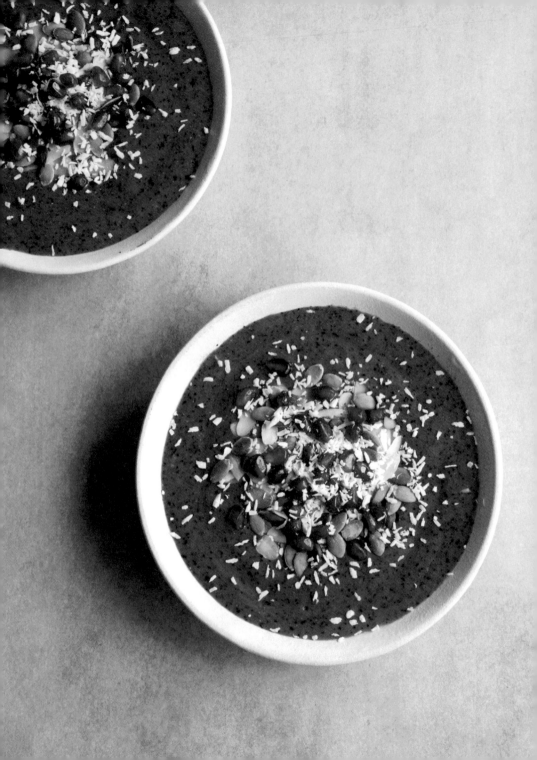

Blueberry-Pom Smoothie Bowl

This blueberry smoothie bowl is a cousin of the açai bowl. With the crunch of pomegranate seeds and sunflower seeds, it's blissfully crunchy and sweet.

Makes 1 serving

10 grams (about 1 tablespoon or scoop) collagen powder

1 tablespoon water

1 cup frozen blueberries

1 frozen banana

½ cup almond milk

¼ to ½ cup pomegranate seeds

1 tablespoon sunflower seeds

Coconut flakes, for garnish

Stir the collagen into 1 tablespoon of the water. Stir well and then transfer the mixture to a blender.

Add the rest of the ingredients and blend well.

Pomegranate is full of catechins, and can help protect skin from UV-B sun damage, while blueberries are packed with resveratrol, antioxidants that have been shown to help prevent aging and help fight inflammation in the body.

Skin-healing superingredient resveratrol simulates the expression of collagen, which makes it vital in healing wounds, and regenerating skin.

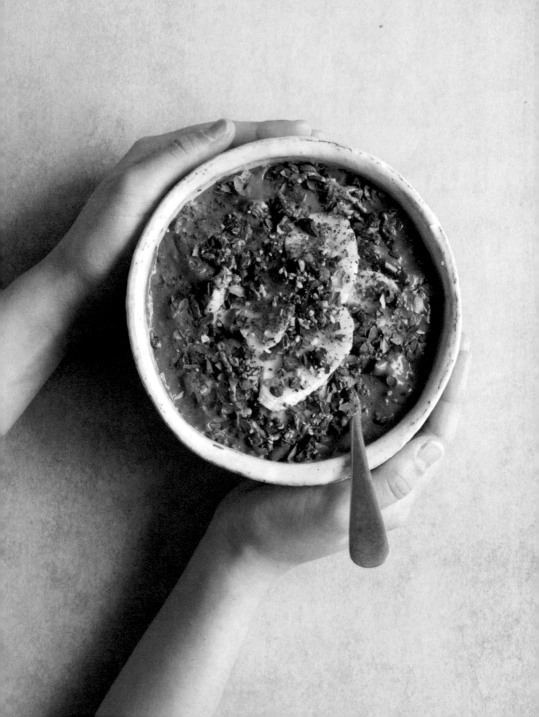

Triple Chocolate Bowl with Almond Butter

Three different kinds of chocolate with cacao-infused nut butter. Need I say more?

Makes 1 serving

10 grams (about 1 tablespoon or scoop) collagen powder

2 teaspoon lucuma powder

3 tablespoons raw cacao powder

½ cup ice

1 frozen banana

1 cup chocolate almond milk

1 tablespoon cacao-infused nut butter

1 to 2 tablespoons stevia chocolate chips

Sliced banana, for garnish (optional)

Place all the ingredients, except the chips, in a blender and blend, adding the almond milk as you go. Add more almond milk or water, based on your desired consistency.

Pour the mixture into a bowl. Mix in the chocolate chips for additional crunch, and also use as a garnish on top, along with banana slices, if using.

TIP

Because this bowl has so many layers of chocolate, it's perfect for adding greens and other vegetables, as the cacao powder, cacao nut butter, and the chocolate almond milk will mask the healthful ingredients that we otherwise wouldn't reach for.

Matcha Mint Chocolate Chip Smoothie Bowl

This smoothie bowl will pleasantly surprise you; not only is it minty fresh, but the kick of matcha adds a boost of energy (and the beautiful, all-natural shade of green). I love having this bowl more as a dessert to substitute for mint chocolate chip ice cream—which happens to be my number-one guilty pleasure and of course, the inspiration for this bowl.

Makes 1 serving

10 grams (about 1 tablespoon or scoop) collagen powder

2 teaspoons matcha powder

2 teaspoons lucuma powder

1 to 2 tablespoons raw cacao pow-der

6 to 8 fresh mint leaves, or 2 drops peppermint oil

½ cup ice

1 frozen banana

1 cup almond milk

1 to 2 tablespoons stevia chocolate chips

Toasted oats, chia seeds, and flaked coconut, for garnish (optional)

Place all the ingredients, except the chips, in a blender and blend, adding the almond milk as you go to reach your desired consistency.

Pour the mixture into a bowl. Mix in the chocolate chips for additional crunch, and also use as a garnish on top, along with toasted oats, chia seeds, and flaked coconut, if using.

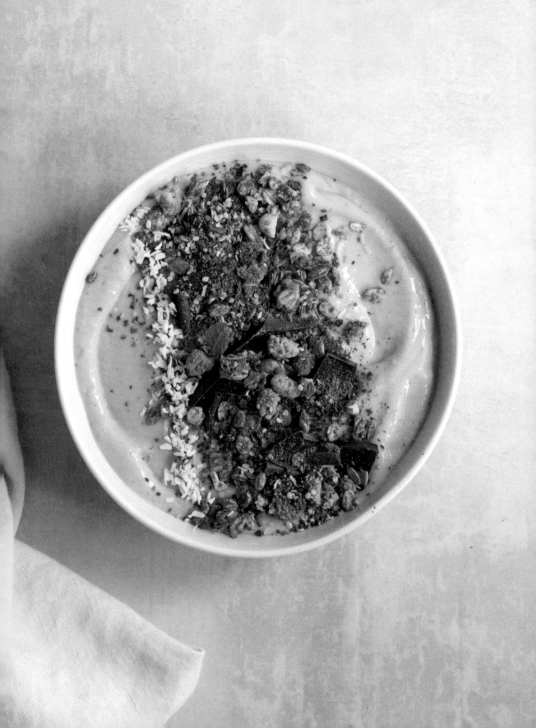

Strawberry Pineapple Banana Bowl

This strawberry banana pineapple bowl is far from basic. And with the sprinkle of coconut flakes and goji berries, you'll have some chewy candied texture to the bowl!

Makes 1 serving

10 grams (about 1 tablespoon or scoop) collagen powder

1 cup frozen strawberries

1 frozen banana

1 cup cubed pineapple

½ cup ice

1 cup of your favorite milk

1 tablespoon goji berries

1 tablespoon coconut flakes

Grated chocolate, for garnish (optional)

Place the collagen powder, frozen strawberries, frozen banana, pineapple, and ice in a blender and blend, adding the almond milk as you go. Add more almond milk or water, based on your desired consistency.

Pour the mixture into a bowl. Sprinkle in the coconut flakes and goji berries before serving Add grated chocolate to garnish, if using.

> Strawberries are a great source of folic acid, a B vitamin that helps regulate DNA repair and synthesis.

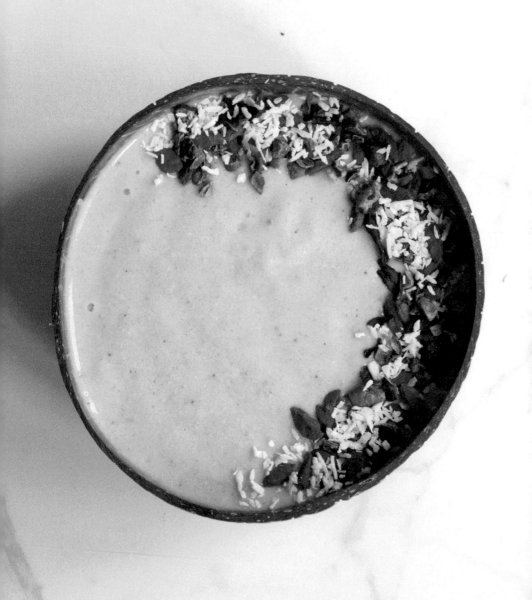

Detox Charcoal Bowl

If you are unfamiliar with activated charcoal—it's the culprit behind this beautiful, intense black of this bowl. But don't let the color throw you off: charcoal is great in flushing out harmful toxins of our body—so turn to this charcoal smoothie bowl for when you need to start your day with a detox. However, because it can also bind to things that aren't so bad for your body, like collagen in this case, I recommend that you still get your daily serving of collagen a few hours after consumption of charcoal.

Makes 1 serving

⅓ cup dry chia seeds

3 cups filtered water

¾ cup frozen blueberries

1 frozen banana

1 cup almond milk

1 teaspoon activated charcoal

Place the chia seeds and water in a bowl. Soak for 20 minutes, then transfer to a blender.

Add all the remaining ingredients and blend together.

Activated charcoal binds to bile like a sponge, and helps remove toxins from our body, and supports our liver and kidney functions by helping excrete these compounds.

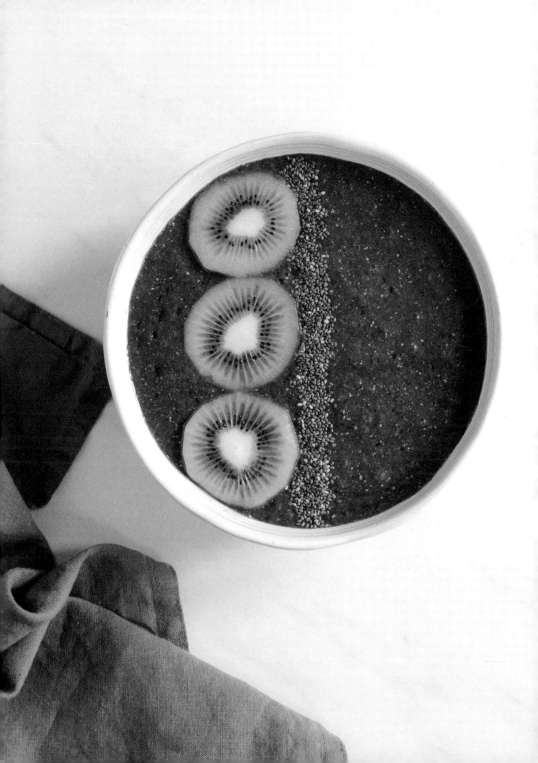

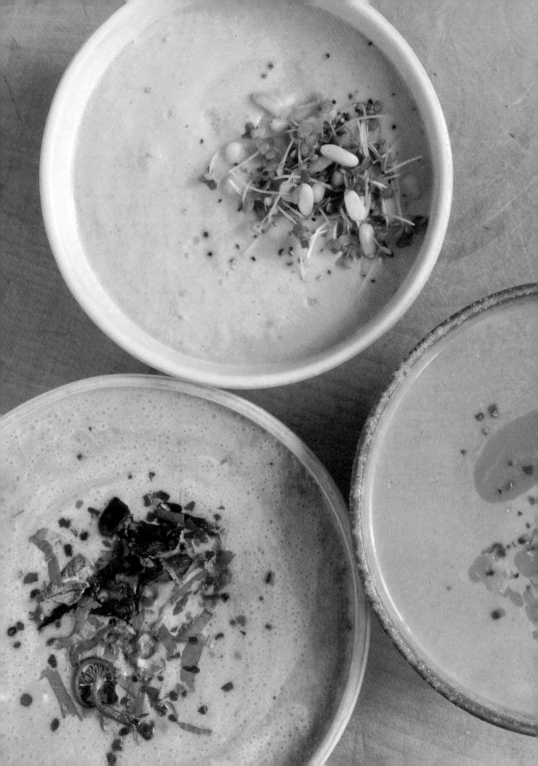

Soups
and Broths

Bone Broth

You didn't think I'd skip the traditional way of consuming collagen, did you?

Makes about 8 cups of bone broth

Bones from a whole chicken (skin and bones from a rotisserie chicken), or beef bones (oxtail, short ribs, or other bones with not much meat attached to them)

Filtered water to cover the bones

1 cup vegetable stock

Fresh herbs, such as parsley or thyme

1 or 2 bay leaves

5 dates

1 tablespoon cider vinegar

4 garlic cloves, peeled

1 white onion

2 large carrots

1 tablespoon coconut oil

Salt and freshly ground black pepper

Place the chicken bones into a 12-quart stockpot, and cover by at least 4 inches with water.

Add the vegetable stock, herbs, bay leaves, dates, vinegar, and garlic.

In a separate pan, sauté the onions and carrots in 1 tablespoon coconut oil until the carrots are soft.

Add the sautéed vegetables to the stockpot. Bring to a low boil (lowest setting).

Simmer for at least 7 hours (more the better).

Strain through cheesecloth, and season with salt and pepper to taste before serving.

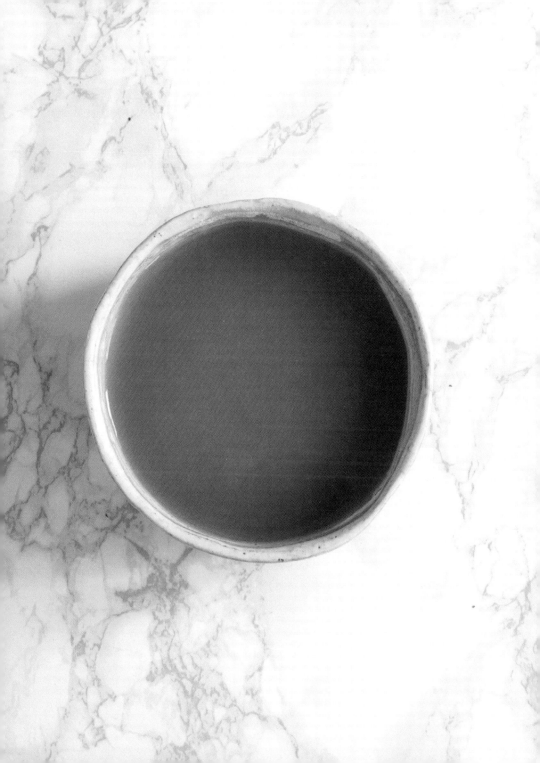

Korean Janchi Soup

This is a miso soup equivalent in the Korean cuisine—this anchovy stock is used as a base for almost every seafood-infused broth. Looking back, this is one of the funniest things my Korean school did. Every day at 3 p.m., parent volunteers would come in to class and hand out three big pieces of anchovies for us to eat, as they are high in protein and packed with collagen and niacin, which are great for your skin and heart health. And as for the word *janchi*? It means "to celebrate"!

Makes 2 to 4 servings

STOCK

6 cups filtered water

2 teaspoons dashima kelp

1 white onion, quartered

25 dried anchovies

1 teaspoon nori (optional)

½ teaspoon Korean chili powder (optional)

Seasoning sauce (recipe follows)

TO MAKE THE STOCK

Bring the water to a boil in a stockpot.

Add the dashima, onion, and anchovies. Simmer for a few minutes.

Add the nori and the chili powder, if using.

Serve with seasoning sauce.

SEASONING SAUCE

1½ tablespoons regular soy sauce

1½ tablespoons rice wine

1 teaspoon sesame oil

1 teaspoon minced garlic

½ teaspoon Korean chili flakes (*gochugaru*)

2 tablespoons finely chopped Asian chives, chives, or green onion

TO MAKE THE SEASONING SAUCE

Mix in a small bowl.

> Dashima is a kelp commonly used to make stock, then thrown away.

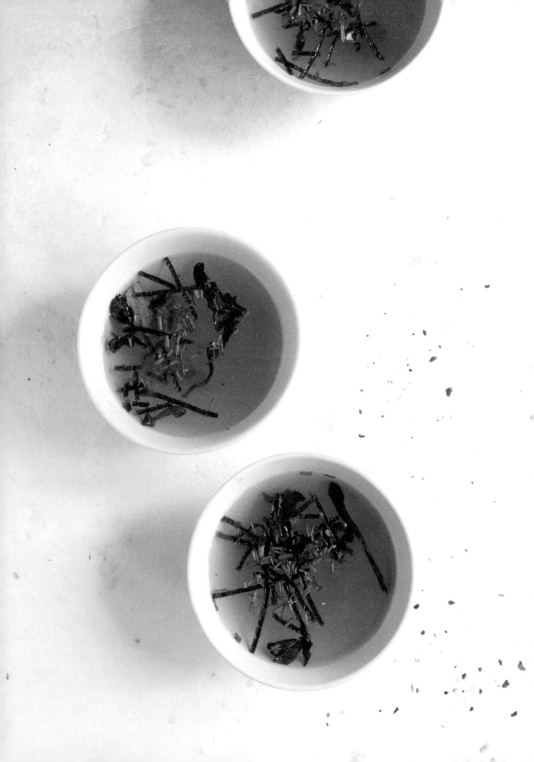

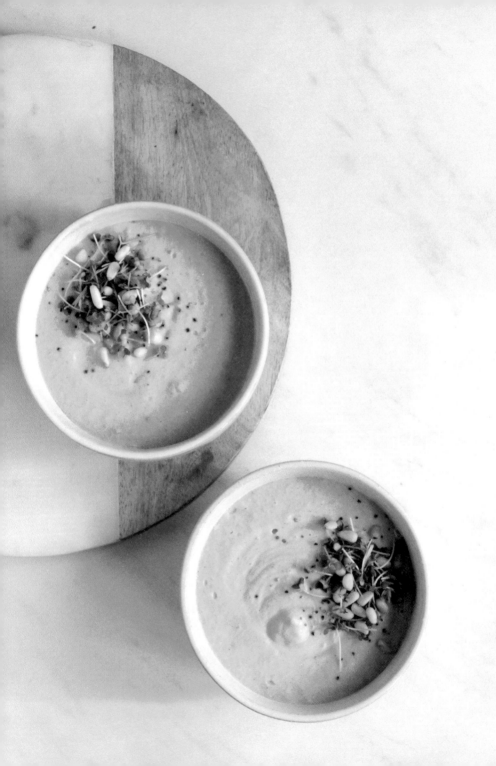

Coconut Butternut Squash Soup

In the wintertime, I often make this soup for my friends and family. It ticks off all the boxes of what makes the perfect soup: rich, creamy, sweet, and savory; but beware, once you make a pot of this, you may eat all of it in less than a day (which isn't so bad, as we are replacing the traditional heavy cream with coconut milk).

Makes 2 to 4 servings

3 tablespoons coconut oil

2 large white onions, finely sliced

1 to 2 garlic cloves, peeled and minced

1 butternut squash

3 cups bone broth (for homemade, see page 122; add additional collagen, if desired)

1 cup coconut milk

1 bay leaf

A pinch each of sea salt and black pepper

Pinch of grated nutmeg

Heat the coconut oil in a skillet and sauté the onions until softened.

Place the onions and all the rest of the ingredients, except the nutmeg, in a slow cooker or stockpot.

Bring to a boil, adding water if need be.

Lower the heat and simmer until the onion quarters become tender and almost disintegrate (but not quite).

Transfer the soup to a blender or food processor (or use an immersion blender) and puree until smooth.

Serve warm with a pinch of nutmeg.

> Butternut squash is packed with fiber, minerals, and vitamins A and C (which I hope that we all know by now is great for our skin).

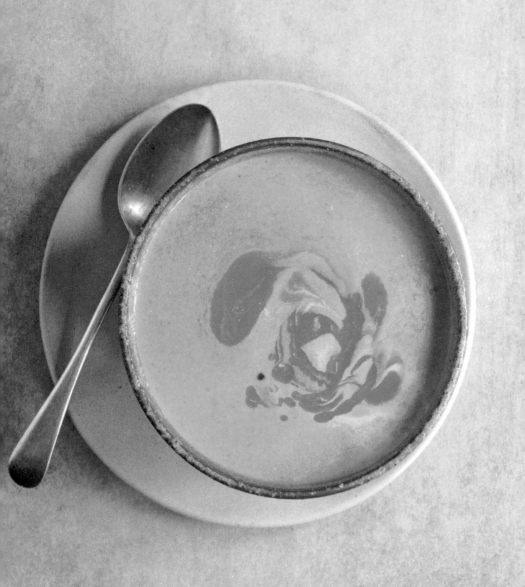

Tomato Bisque Soup

Koreans put garlic into just about anything, so I grew up being very fond of garlic. Garlic always adds the umami to soups and bisques: and when combined with coconut cream, its flavor comes out even better!

Makes 2 to 4 servings

1 tablespoon coconut oil

3 garlic cloves, peeled

1 white onion

6 plum tomatoes

1 teaspoon thyme

1 teaspoon oregano

1 cup coconut milk

2 cups diced fresh tomatoes

2 cups bone broth (for homemade, see page 122; add additional collagen, if desired)

10 fresh basil leaves

2 bay leaves

One 14-ounce can unsweetened coconut cream

Salt and freshly ground black pepper

Heat the coconut oil in a large saucepan over medium heat.

Add the garlic and onion and sauté until the onion has softened and has become translucent.

Add the plum tomatoes with thyme, oregano, coconut milk, and sauté until the tomato peels have disintegrated.

Transfer the mixture to a stockpot and add the diced tomatoes, bone broth, basil, and bay leaves.

Simmer for 30 minutes over medium heat.

Blend the soup with an immersion blender until smooth. Stir in coconut cream and warm if necessary.

Season to taste with salt and pepper.

Green Thai Curry

This is actually the exact recipe I was making when I got burned, so be careful! But no matter how painful the memory of creating it two years ago, this is one of my favorites to this day.

Makes 2 servings

2 garlic cloves, peeled and minced

3 tablespoons Thai green curry paste

1 cup bone broth (for homemade, see page 122; add extra collagen powder, if desired)

½ peeled sweet potato, diced

½ Asian eggplant, peeled and diced

One 14-ounce can coconut milk

Asian fish sauce to taste (optional)

Rice vinegar to taste (optional)

Sesame oil, for serving

Chopped scallions, for garnish

Freshly squeezed lime juice, for serving

Add bone broth, sweet potato, and eggplant to the pot and bring to a simmer over medium-high heat. Simmer until vegetables are soft, about 15 minutes. Blend the soup with an immersion blender until smooth. Stir in coconut milk and warm again but don't allow the soup to boil.

Stir in fish sauce and vinegar, if using.

To serve, pour into bowls, drizzle with sesame oil, sprinkle with scallions and squeeze with lime juice.

Compounds found in curry can have anti-inflammatory properties—however, too much spice could negatively impact you as well, so make sure you taste as you go!

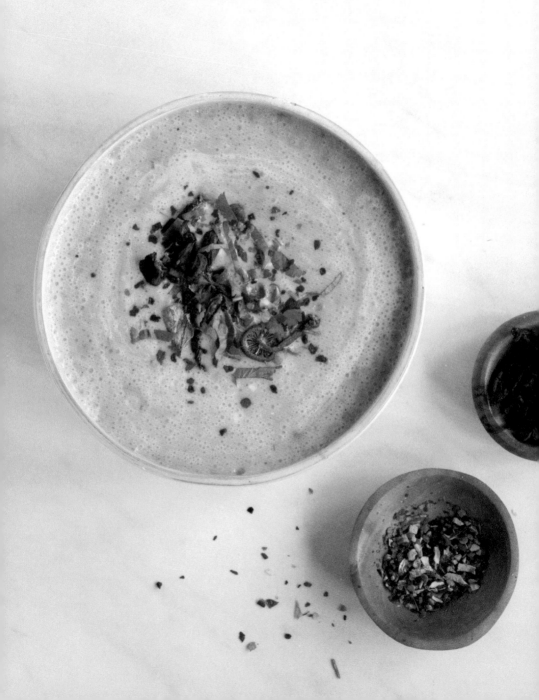

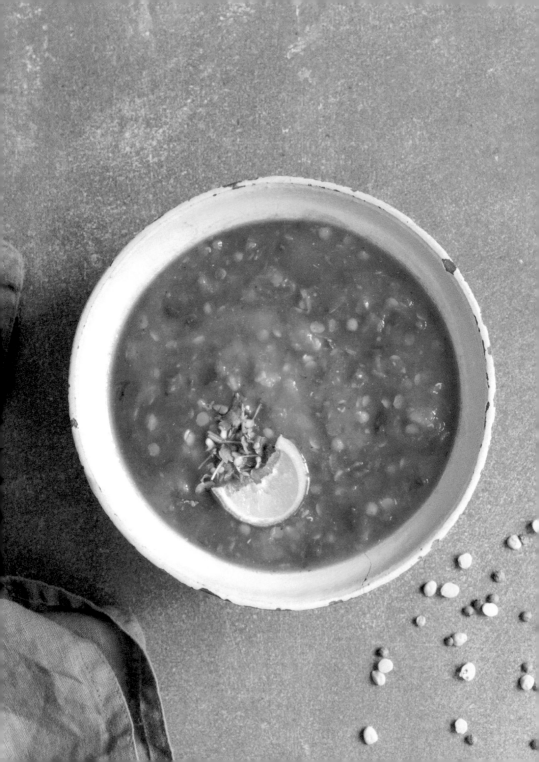

Turmeric Carrot Lentil Soup

This soup is perfect to make on a Sunday night, to have in your fridge throughout the week. I like to take it to work as well, and reach for it as my afternoon snack—I love that it keeps me full for hours, especially with all of the protein derived from the lentils (on top of the collagen)!

Makes 4 servings

4 cups low-sodium vegetable stock

2 teaspoons thyme

2 bay leaves

40 grams (about 4 tablespoons or scoops) collagen powder

2 teaspoon ground turmeric

1 cup dried red lentils, rinsed

1 tablespoon coconut oil

1 sweet white onion, diced

3 carrots, diced

Salt and pepper

Freshly squeezed lemon juice

Combine the vegetable stock, thyme, bay leaves, collagen, and turmeric in a large stockpot. Bring to a boil, then add the lentils.

Lower the heat to medium, and cook for 15 to 20 minutes.

When the lentils are almost fully cooked (about 10 minutes in), heat the coconut oil in a separate pan.

Add the diced onion and carrots to the pan and sauté until softened.

Add the sautéed vegetables to the stockpot and stir with the lentils. Simmer for another 5 minutes.

Add salt and pepper and a spritz of lemon juice to taste.

Protein-dense lentils contain phytochemicals and antioxidants that can help lower blood pressure, improve heart health, and reduce risk for cardiovascular diseases.

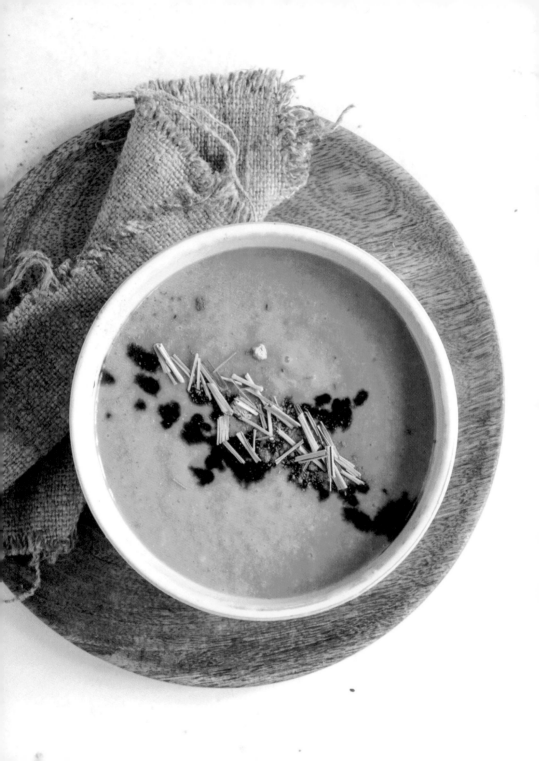

Apple Onion Bisque

With a mix of both apples and onions, this soup is a perfect mix of decadent and healthy.

Makes 4 servings

1 tablespoon coconut oil

3 large yellow onions, finely sliced

2 garlic cloves, peeled and minced

6 cups vegetable stock

40 grams (about 4 tablespoons or scoops) collagen powder

2 red apples, peeled, cored, and cubed

1 cup organic applesauce

½ cup apple cider

One 14-ounce can coconut milk

Salt and pepper

Chopped chives, for garnish

Heat the coconut oil in a large saucepan over medium-high heat. Sauté the onions and garlic until they soften and become tender.

Transfer the mixture to a stockpot and add the vegetable stock and collagen powder. Let simmer over medium heat for 30 minutes.

Sauté the cubed apples in a skillet over medium-high heat, then add to the simmering soup. Add the applesauce and cider.

Blend with an immersion blender until smooth.

Add the coconut milk, and warm if necassary. Season to taste with salt and pepper.

Garnish with chives.

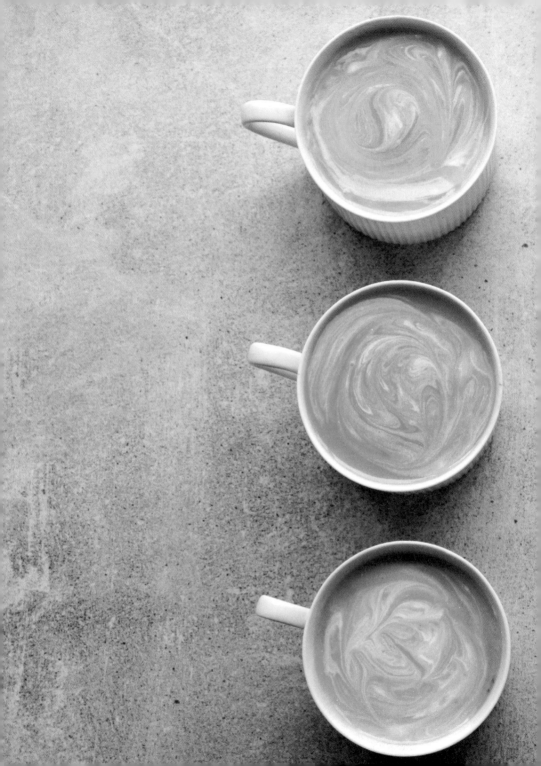

Collagen
Boot Camp

THE 10 KOREAN SKINCARE TIPS MY GRANDMOTHER PASSED DOWN TO ME

My skincare regimen—both external and internal—all come from my Korean roots—more specifically, my grandmother.

My grandmother is an amazing chef—she escaped from North Korea, and to make ends meet and survive, she started her own restaurant in Seoul, where food was scarce, and people had to turn to every part of the animal as well as obscure plants from both land and sea to satiate themselves. Nothing was ever thrown out (she used to tell me that people would even fight over who would eat the eyeballs of fish), so she had to get creative with using every formidable bit of an ingredient.

She also took the "overfeed your grandchildren" to a new level (though I'm not complaining, by any means). It was one of her biggest signs of affection when, after taking the bones out of the fish, she would chopstick over a chunk of the grilled fish, skin on, onto my bowl of piping hot rice, instead of eating it herself. (In Korea, since everyone knows all of the "good stuff," a.k.a. the collagen, is in the fish of the skin, it was quite the symbol of her love when she would give it away.)

She is a culinary genius, who knows everything there is to know about every fruit, every vegetable. I was lucky that she raised me (in Korea, grandparents often live with their eldest child and babysit the grandchildren), as she is my first gateway to understanding nutrition. She taught me everything I know about food, its magical superpowers, and how eating one thing can affect me positively, or negatively, for the rest of the day.

She inadvertently trained me to keep to this holistic, 360-degree lifestyle that all circles back to maintaining a healthy, glowing skin. Whether or not I realized it when I was a child, I am so grateful that I have unknowingly been practicing this Korean skincare "diet" all these years.

I still keep these rules close to my heart today:

RULE #1. STAY HYDRATED, AND DRINK LOTS OF FILTERED WATER AND TEA. LOTS OF IT.

This may be the most important rule of all. Growing up, I drank *only* filtered water. It was unheard of to drink from the tap (really, every household in South Korea has the kind of water purification machine that you only see in doctor's offices here in the States), so my fridge was always filled with pints and pints of the highest-quality water. Often, there are radicals in unfiltered water that bother our system, and therefore our skin—so, don't risk it—always go with filtered!

For your skin to look dewy and glowing, it needs to be hydrated at the cellular level. Usually, dry skin is caused by dehydration of the body or malnourishment of certain fats. So, remembering to drink throughout the day is really important.

Barley Tea

Growing up, my fridge was always filled with pints of barley tea. You can't go to any Korean restaurant without being served plentiful cupfuls of this golden liquid. Barley tea is great for you, from head to toe: it is known to improve blood circulation, which is great for your skin. You can drink barley tea hot or cold.

To make a pitcher of roasted barley tea, add 2 to 3 tablespoons of roasted barley to 4 cups of boiling water. Allow the grains to simmer for 5 to 10 minutes before straining out the kernels. For a nutritional bonus, let the kernels rest, then eat them once they've softened. To make cold barley tea, simply put a pitcher in the fridge, or add 1 to 2 tablespoons of barley kernels to 4 cups of water and let it sit overnight.

RULE #2. REST, RELAX, AND SLEEP AS MUCH AS YOU CAN.
Give yourself breaks from difficult, strenuous environments once in a while. When we are emotionally challenged, our skin will naturally reflect that exact state. And the best way to do this? Sleep. My grandmother always had a makeshift bed in her living room for me. During this restorative stage of sleep, our blood pressure drops, breathing slows down, blood flow moves to the muscles, and our tissue is repaired. Our body releases growth hormones during this stage as

well—hormones essential for growth and development, including muscle development.

RULE #3. USE BOTANICALS AND OTHER FOODS TO HELP WITH HEALING.

Koreans love ancient medicine, and often turn to botanicals (roots, herbs, even fruits), or botanical-based teas, for healing. You will find examples throughout this book.

Matcha for Health

Turn to matcha over coffee for that extra kick of caffeine: matcha contains L-theanine, a mental focus stimulant, which provides a natural punch of caffeine without the crash (that coffee is usually accompanied by). Matcha is also a great source of these antiaging antioxidants called catechins, which support your liver's detoxification process, while the overload of caffeine from coffee can stress out your liver even more. Green tea can also prevent enzyme activity that breaks down collagen.

RULE #4. EAT GOLGORU: DON'T BE PICKY WITH FOOD, AND HAVE AS MUCH KIMCHI, FISH, AND BROTH AS POSSIBLE.

We all know that feeling when we feel too bloated from eating the wrong foods, and how the next day, our skin seems to take a hit. But those same problems could occur if we are not eating the *right* foods. Which is why we should always ensure that we are eating a variety of foods (a.k.a. to eat *golgoru*). This term was probably uttered at every meal my grandmother made me.

One of her favorite things to push at me was kimchi. Kimchi, a fermented, pickled cabbage iconic to our culture, is dense with minerals, vitamins A, B, and C, fat-free, and most important, loaded with probiotics.

RULE #5. CHOOSE FRUITS OVER DESSERTS HIGH IN SUGAR CONTENT.

At the end of every meal, Koreans eat apples, tangerines, Korean pears, and watermelon for dessert. We rarely eat cookies, bread, or cake—I never knew what a chocolate chip cookie or peanut butter jelly sandwich was until I moved to California at the age of ten.

Once in a while, Koreans indulge in bread, usually in the form of a small pastry.

RULE #6. NOTHING SALTY AFTER EIGHT P.M.

Your body will not be able to excrete salt during your eight hours of sleep, and you can retain water.

RULE #7. NEVER FORGET TO SEH-SU (A LITERAL DEFINITION IS "WASHING OF THE FACE").

Again, my grandmother didn't ever push the 10-step regimen at me or any of my siblings, while we were growing up. But what she did strictly enforce is the seh-su. She always told me, "Think of all of the dirt and residue that is sitting on your skin after a day in this polluted city. Do you want to all those dirt bugs in your pillowcase?" (I may never go to sleep peacefully again, but this is probably my most effective reminder.)

RULE #8. EXFOLIATE ALL YOUR DEAD SKIN CELLS (DDEH) AWAY.

I grew up attending communal bathhouses with my aunts and mothers, where we would dedicate a whole day receiving hammams (a.k.a. Turkish baths), spending hours in saunas, and getting our skin exfoliated professionally with these viscose fabric mitts (the traditional, old-school version of the electronic brushes that we use today). Koreans take exfoliating to another level: we call the residual, dead skin cells ddeh, and once in a while, will scrub our skin raw—from head to toe—to make sure that we have shed our outermost layer. When I moved to Los Angeles, and realized that this was not a regular activity in the States, I was so shocked.

RULE #9. SUNBLOCK, SUNBLOCK, SUNBLOCK. OR PARASOL.

Koreans are probably the only human beings that wear hats, scarves, and long gloves in 100 degree-plus, boiling hot weather—and not because we get cold so easily, but because we are trying to protect our skin. We don't go anywhere without applying sunblock, even on rainy days; we sometimes cancel plans and don't even go outside if it's too hot, solely for the reason that it may be too damaging to our skin. And what do we use if there are no winter apparel to prevent the UV radiation? Parasols.

RULE #10. LISTEN TO YOUR SKIN.

Koreans often look to a person's complexion to deduce someone's overall health or emotional state—and it makes complete sense why: our skin is among the first organs to reflect any signs of nutritional deficiencies or imbalance. We can often tell what's going at the cellular level when we study the condition of our skin. It's a totally acceptable question to ask, "Why does your skin look like that?"—not because we condone rude comments, but because our health conditions can be truly reflected in our skin.

SALLY'S FAVORITE FOODS TO EAT EVERY DAY

Here are a few of my personal favorite foods that I try to eat every day.

For specific amounts, please consult with a nutritionist or your doctor—some of these foods, such as shrimp, could be harmful to those who struggle with heart diseases, as shellfish is high in cholesterol.

WHERE YOU CAN FIND SKIN-HEALING NUTRIENTS

CIDER VINEGAR (ACETIC ACID) The acetic acid in vinegar has been shown to assist with weight loss due to its ability to inhibit lipogenesis (the formation of fat cells), which is known to lower both waist size and BMI. Maintaining the skin pH below 5.5 is vital for suppressing the growth of microbes that cause pathological skin infections, including Staphylococcus aureus. The acidity of the skin is essential for enhancing the antimicrobial barrier. Many people use cider vinegar as a way to keep the pH low.

GARLIC (ALLICIN) Allicin, found in garlic, can have immune system-supporting traits that fight the common cold. Diallyl disulfide, also found in garlic, helps inhibit histone deacetylases, which has shown to treat osteoar-thritis. Sulfur baths, along with other sulfur treatments, may help treat acne, rosacea, psoriasis, eczema, dan-druff, and discolored skin patches.

GREEN TEA (CATECHINS AND L-THEANINE) Catechins are found in tea extracts. They have antioxidant func-tions in the body.

One of the most well-known catechins is called EGCG for short, and it's especially great for skin. In one study, EGCG did wonders for ugly-looking keloid scars by making them shrink, slicing the keloid mast cells that cause inflammation—by 98%—and stopping the buildup of new blood vessels to feed the keloid scar. EGCG reduces the collagen types I and III of protein, makes the keloid cells die, and decreases the production of the keloid cell.

GOTU KOLA HERB (CENTELLA ASIATICA) Reinforces the skin-rejuvenation matrix to make it more dense, using collagen and fibronectin proteins

RAW CACAO, MUSHROOMS, AND BLUEBERRIES (CHRO-MIUM) For skin to start healing, there needs to be a balance of cell reproduction and differentiation of blood cells. Chromium balances sugar levels so keratinocytes in the epidermis and fibroblasts in the dermis can be created in balanced ratios to facilitate healing.

SEAWEED (COENZYME Q10) Reverses sun damage of skin by increasing the fibroblast count; promotes syn-thesis of collagen/elastin; reduces collagenase, which destroys collagen, while reducing spots in the skin; also preserves the mitochondrial function so cells can act as an antioxidant.

COFFEE (COFFEE POLYPHENOLS) Improves skin's barrier functions in addition to circulation, especially in dry skin. A better pH level in skin is achieved with more fats on the outer layer of the skin.

ANCHOVY STOCK (COLLAGEN)

TURMERIC AND GREEN CURRY (CURCUMIN) Found in turmeric, curcumin prohibits the inflammatory agent PhK that is usually triggered by injuries to the body, including the damage done by the sun. Curcumin increases collagen synthesis and cell proliferation that allows faster wound healing. It also improves bone health by modulating enzymes and proteins responsible for bone remodeling.

RAW CACAO (EPICATECHIN) Epicatechin increases levels of follistatin to build maintain muscles and fight the myostatin protein that limits muscle growth.

SOY, GLYCINE MAX (FOR GENISTEIN) Genistein, found in soy, has proven beauty benefits that include collagen stimulation, antioxidant properties, lightening of the skin, and anti-inflammation. Genistein has also been shown to help rejuvenate the strength of skin in women during their postmenopausal years, and it has been associated with improved elasticity, and sun damage recovery.

GINGER (GINGEROLS AND SHOGAOLS) Ginger consumption has been shown to assist with arthritis pains, nausea, and reduction of muscle pains by inhibiting leokotrienes, which cause inflammation.

SHRIMP AND SHELLFISH EXOSKELETONS (GLUCOSAMINE) Glucosamine is essential in the synthesis of hyaluronate and proteoglycans, both essential to the formation of connective tissues and the aging of the body. Hyaluroate increases have led to the improvement of skin structure and hydration levels.

CORDYCEPS (GLUTHATHIONE) Cordyceps has glutathione, which is known to help reduce inflammation and treat liver and heart disease; Cordyceps also regulates L-carnitine, critical for energy metabolism and liver recovery.

SPIRULINA, EGGS, RED MEATS, APRICOTS, AND BLACK-STRAP MOLASSES (IRON) Iron is essential for healthy skin, mucous membranes, hair, and nails. Deficiency causes symptoms of malnourishment along with slower healing of wounds and inflammation.

RED VEGETABLES, TOMATOES, RED PEPPERS, BEETS, AND WATERMELON (LYCOPENE) Lycopene is the natural carotenoid found in tomatoes and red vegatables. Increased lycopene consumption has shown to reduce seborrhea, yield better skin pH, increase skin density, and higher counts of collagen and elastic fibers. It has also been shown to protect against the development of redness in skin after sun exposure.

ALMONDS, CASHEWS, SOY, FERMENTED FOODS, SUCH AS TEMPEH, SWEET POTATOES, AND SPIRULINA, DARK LEAFY GREENS, SUCH AS KALE, SPINACH, AND SWISS CHARD (MAGNESIUM) Magnesium, most commonly found in nuts, is a key catalyst in producing hyaluronic acid. So, if there doesn't exist enough of magnesium, production of hyaluronic acid may be stalled. Magnesium is also needed for DNA/RNA synthesis and the reproduction and protein synthesis in all cells, including skin cells.

FATTY FISH, SUCH AS TUNA, COD, SALMON, MACKEREL, AND KRILL (OMEGA-3 FATTY ACIDS) Generally, there are 2 different types of omega-3 fatty acids: EPA and DHA. EPA increases number of collagen and elastin fibers in aged skin. EPA helps the permeability of the membranes protect from foreign substances and toxins. If you are not a fan of salmon, try tuna, cod, mackerel, and krill as your first substitutes to salmon for omega-3 consumption.

AÇAI (POLYPHENOLS) Polyphenols can improve memory and assist in weight loss; they may also help lower cholesterol levels.

BANANA (POTASSIUM) Potassium, generally found in

bananas, can improve heart health and may lower the risk of stroke.

KIMCHI AND YOGURT (PROBIOTICS) Probiotics have been shown to benefit skin troubled with inflammation and dermatitis. The Lactobacillus group of bacteria are known to prevent certain forms of skin disease and improve a number of skin conditions. Oral supplements of Lactobacillus in animals has been shown to help fight sun damage.

JAPANESE KNOTWEED HERB (POLYGONUM CUSPIDA-TUM), RED WINE, GRAPE SKINS, ROOTS OF WHITE HELLE-BORE (VERATRUM GRANDIFLORUM), SKIN OF PEANUTS, AND BERRIES (RESVERATROL) Resveratrol is a potent scavenger of free radicals, making it an antioxidant/antiaging molecule. It has been used to treat inflammation, arthritis, and gout. It helps strengthen cartilage. Wound healing is also catalyzed by resveratrol, achieved by improving blood circulation and recovery effects on the skin. Particular studies have shown that resveratrol improved the severity of wrinkles and fine lines. Resveratrol has increased overall skin thickness by substantial amounts over continued application balanced with vitamin E. It also extends the life of collagen by preventing the creation of enzymes that break collagen down.

WHEAT GERM, SEAFOOD, SUCH AS TUNA AND SALMON, GARLIC, BRAZIL NUTS, EGGS, BROWN RICE, AND WHOLE WHEAT BREAD (SELENIUM) Selenium is an antioxidant that contributes to tissue elasticity by preventing or minimalizing cell damage from free radicals. In addition to neutralizing peroxides from damaging the skin, selenium also helps protect the skin from UV light damage.

GARLIC, ONIONS, AND HIGH-QUALITY ANIMAL PROTEINS (SULFUR) Different applications of sulfur can help treat such skin disorders as acne, rosacea, psoriasis, eczema, dandruff, folliculitis, warts, and skin conditions of discoloration, as well as arthritis.

OYSTERS, BLACK BEANS, AND DARK MEAT ON CHICKEN AND TURKEY (ZINC) Both a mineral and antioxidant, zinc minimalizes oxidative damage to the skin. Also removes free radicals from superoxides and -OH groups that come from the metals iron and copper.

WHERE YOU CAN FIND SKIN-HEALING VITAMINS

VITAMIN A Can be found in both animal and plant foods. Vitamin A is crucial for vision, immunity, red blood cell synthesis, reproduction, bone cell metabolism, maintenance of mucosal tissues, and fighting inflammation. The strength of bonds between cells and the growth of cells are both dependent upon vitamin A. Deficiency can lead to extreme dryness of the skin in addition to extra shedding of skin cells at an abnormal rate.

- Cow's milk
- Cheese
- Eggs
- Chicken
- Shrimp
- Fish: cod, tuna, sardines, salmon, and halibut
- Scallops
- Yogurt
- Fish liver and fish liver oil, and livers of sheep, beef, and other large animals
- Carotenoids: primarily orange and dark green vegetables such as carrots, sweet potatoes, pumpkin, kale, spinach, broccoli, mustard greens, parsley, turnip greens, beet greens, bell peppers, and cantaloupe (although these are beta-carotene, the precursor of vitamin A).

VITAMIN B, NIACINAMIDE (B3) BIOTIN (B7), FOLIC ACID/ FOLATE (B9), B12 B vitamins play the role of maintaining the skin's equilibrium. Vitamin B3 is an important antioxidant for the skin due to its small size that allows it to permeate through skin to regulate cell metabolism and regeneration. Nicotinamide, the active form of vitamin B3, has anti-inflammatory, antioxidant, and immunomodulatory functions, while stimulating skin cells to regenerate. The use of nicotinamide in one animal case study has shown to create more blood vessels and collagen within the area of treatment. Its topical use has also shown to help wrinkles paired with better skin elasticity. Biotin is closely related with vitamin B12 metabolism and digestion, and the overall process leads to DNA synthesis and detoxification of the body. Folic acid, the B vitamin linked with DNA repair and synthesis, is constantly needed to fight UV exposure and sun damage. The lack of folic acid or deficiency of it can lead to increased chances of skin cancer.

- Oysters provide a low-calorie option and a long list of health benefits.
- Biotin food sources include egg yolk, liver, and yeast.
- Folic acid is found in the following foods: broccoli, green leafy vegetables, beans, peas, grapefruit, orange juice, cantaloupe, liver, other organ meats, and fortified cereals.
- Vitamin B12 is naturally found in animal products, including fish, meat, poultry, eggs, milk, and milk products.

VITAMIN C Hesperidin, found in oranges, can improve heart health while preventing kidney stones by decreasing urinary saturation of calcium oxalate. Vitamin C also helps amino acids convert to collagen, while antioxidant vitamin C is water-soluble and reduces levels of free radicals linked with aging of the skin. Also increases moisture of the skin through increases in collagen synthesis.

- Citrus fruits: oranges, limes, lemons, and grapefruits
- Acerola berry
- Rose hips
- The herb camu-camu

VITAMIN E Vitamin E is an antioxidant known to lower inflammation by decreasing prostaglandin production. Promotes immune functions by replicating T cells. Vitamin E removes free radicals, but the supply of it can be immediately depleted by one dose of sun exposure. Vitamin E and other antioxidants help maintain homeostasis by protecting the proteins and fats in the skin from oxidation. Topical use of vitamin E has shown to maintain moisture better while protecting the skin from sun damage at the same time. Vitamin E combined with C has shown to provide a synergy effect to fight redness and sun damage. Although vitamin E deficiency is rare in humans, deficiency in animals have shown to result in the breakdown of collagen structure.

- Spinach
- Seeds and nuts

30-DAY CHALLENGE: THE 30-DAY KOREAN SKINCARE DIET

America's obsession with beauty, and antiaging, is overrated. Aging isn't a crime, it's an inevitable, natural process, and beauty exists in all ages and forms.

However, that's easier said than done. And the truth is, our insecurities around skin—whether it be from aging, or cellulite, or acne—are problems that get in the way of our day-to-day activities, problems that weigh us down. But what if I told you that those are probably problems that you could solve, prevent, or at the very least ameliorate, with a healthier lifestyle and diet? And that instead of covering up these problems, we can solve them at the core?

Because it's true. Most of those problems are directly correlated to what's happening underneath our skin (such as our declining supply of collagen) and can be combated with a thoughtful diet and regimen. Especially when it comes to fighting the symptoms of aging.

But I know that all of this could seem intimidating, maybe even too complex, to someone who may be new to the world of ingestible skincare—which is why I've designed a 30-day lifestyle guide for you, designed with the purpose of driving you to healthier eating habits that incorporate collagen, our essential building blocks for skin, as well as what guards you against skin-impacting health conditions, such as inflammation, indigestion, and fatigue.

However, most people are unaware of the fact that many of their most stubborn skin and hair problems start at the root of nutrition and biology—and turn to covering up their problems, instead of solving them at the core. And when it comes to fighting the symptoms of aging, this couldn't be truer.

But remember, everything starts at the cellular level. And because it takes about four weeks for the surface of our skin to renew and our cells to turn over, be patient.* Hair transformations take longer: results can take six months to a year.

So, using a recipe a day, I challenge you to the "Clean Skin Korean Diet" Boot Camp—a program combining Korean skincare rituals passed down to me from my grandmother, mother, and aunts, with the research I've amassed since being burned. But don't worry: the focus of this program is less extreme eliminations of food groups, and more about shifting your daily lifestyle to incorporate skin-friendly foods and mindful habits that Koreans have ingrained into their day to day.

A TYPICAL DAY WOULD LOOK LIKE THIS

Every day, wake up to a simple collagen-packed drink before breakfast.

For breakfast, turn to a healthy balance of fats and carbohydrates, such as an avocado toast that includes a gluten-free, multigrain slice of toast. Avoid pastries, breads, jams, and butter.

For lunch, turn to steamed fish, such as salmon; some roots and vegetables; and a cup of brown rice. Steaming eliminates the need for oil and butter, while salmon contains healthy fats that are integral in keeping your skin plump and soft.

For dinner, exercise portion control, and be the pickiest you can be: stay as far as you can from fried foods, sugary desserts, and dairy-based drinks.

---

* According to *Radical Beauty: How to Transform Yourself from the Inside Out,* by Deepak Chopra and Kimberly Snyder (2016).

Koreans do not have restrictive diets—although many of us are generally gluten-free and lactose-intolerant, we generally do not cut out any food groups entirely. However, we do exercise portion control, and say no to junk foods on many occasions.

My rule of thumb here is to not consume anything "white" very often. White is an unnatural color for food: sugar, flour, cheese, and milk. And stay away from man-made and processed foods as much as you can; long story short, they're bad for you—from head to toe.

In addition:

- Eat lots of different and colorful veggies.
- Get your healthy fats from salmon, avocados, and nuts. Fat is not evil! It's actually essential for beauty and optimal skin; however, the source of the fat matters. Try to stick with plant-based and nutrient-dense seeds, nuts, and avocados.
- Stay away from what upsets your stomach: junk food, oily foods, alcohol, and cigarettes.
- Lastly, don't forget that it's always about balance.

Despite ritualizing the most perfect diet, our skin and hair need care and attention from the outside as well. Just not the crazy complex routine you're thinking.

It's also often an impossible feat, and downright tiring, trying to check off all the boxes when it comes to "what we need to do," but this is about balance—balance of your outside with what is happening within. Because even if you take one component seriously, such as purchasing the most high-quality moisturizers and eye creams, without internal nourishment, your skin will still struggle. And of course, if you have compromised digestion, or are under constant emotional stress, no amount of collagen, antioxidants, vitamins, and high-quality moisturizers will do the trick.

ACKNOWLEDGMENTS

I would like to express my gratitude to my grandmother, who raised me and taught me everything I know.

Also, thanks to:
Dr. Tess Mauricio, for her research and enthusiastic foreword,
Ann Triestman and Aurora Bell, for their patient guidance,
Jo Harding, for her beautiful photography,
Brigitte Kozena, for her photo styling advice,
Mia Adorante, for inspiring me to contribute my Korean Diet
story to *W Magazine*—the piece that started it all,
and the Crushed Tonic community, for endless support.

Finally, I wish to thank:
my mother, Sunny, and my father, Casey, for pushing me to always
give my all,
my Aunt Micha and Uncle Norman, my biggest cheerleaders,
my sister, Christine, for never doubting my passion,
my brother, Billy, for being my pillar wherever and whenever,
and my friends and mentors for their love and encouragement
throughout my process.

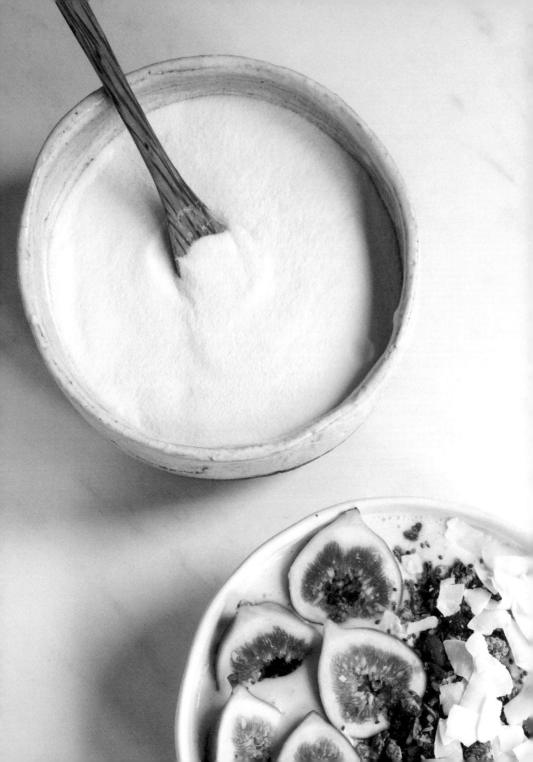

COLLAGEN IN SKIN

www.ncbi.nlm.nih.gov/pmc/articles/PMC4685482/pdf/jmf.2015.0022.pdf

In 2015, researchers from France, Belgium, and Japan found that in their two placebo-controlled clinical trials of daily collagen supplementation for eight weeks, skin hydration improved significantly after eight weeks, while the dermal layer of the skin increased significantly after only four weeks. Both of these effects from the collagen supplement lasted more than 12 weeks.

In another study, a hydrolyzed collagen supplemental drink also containing hyaluronic acid and essential vitamins and minerals given to postmenopausal women had antiaging properties. The women showed significant and positive effects on skin wrinkling, elasticity, and hydration.

For cellulite: Collagen supplements may also help improve the appearance of cellulite. In a German and Brazilian study in 2015, doctors gave 105 women who had moderate amounts of cellulite an oral supplement of 2.5 bioactive collagen peptides over the course of six months. At the end of that period, the women's dermal skin layer had greater density, and they had a significant reduction in cellulite and in waviness in their thighs. The effects were more pronounced in women who were not overweight.

COLLAGEN IN HAIR

Because it contains the amino acid methionine, collagen may improve the appearance of your hair and nails and, possibly, even decrease hair loss. In one study of 30 people with hair loss, in which one group received a preparation of amino acids together with a Vitamin B complex, and the other group received a placebo, the portion of hair in the growth phase was 10 percent higher in the methionine group than in the placebo group after half a year.

155

COLLAGEN FOR SLEEP

Because collagen contains the amino acid glycine, collagen may help reduce insomnia. Doctors tested the effects of taking a supplement containing 3 grams of glycine on insomnia patients. The supplement reportedly reduced their fatigue and sleepiness during the next day.

COLLAGEN FOR JOINTS

In one randomized, controlled trial on the efficacy of a collagen supplement, Spanish researchers found that when 250 volunteers with knee arthtritis were given a 10-gram collagen supplement daily for six months, their arthritis pain improved. The people who had the worst arthritis and ate the least amount of meat regularly experienced the greatest reduction in pain.

REFERENCES FOR NECESSARY NUTRIENTS

ACETIC ACID

Elias, P. M. "The Skin Barrier as an Innate Immune Element." *Semin Immunopathol* 29 (2007): 3–14.

Park, K. "Role of Micronutrients in Skin Health and Function." *Biomol Ther (Seoul)* 23, no. 3 (May 2015): 207–17. https://www.ncbi.nlm.nih.gov/pmc/articles/PMC4428712/.

CATECHINS

Bickers, D. R., and M. Athar. "Oxidative Stress in the Pathogenesis of Skin Disease." *J Invest Dermatol* 126 (2006): 2565–75. https://www.ncbi.nlm.nih.gov/pubmed/17108903.

Syed, F., et al. "Ex Vivo Evaluation of Antifibrotic Compounds in Skin Scarring: EGCG and Silencing of PAI-1 Independently Inhibit Growth and Induce Keloid Shrinkage." *Lab Invest* 93, no. 8 (August 2013): 946–60. doi: 10.1038/labinvest.2013.82. Epub July 8, 2013.

CENTELLA ASIATICA

Hashim, P. "The Effect of Centella asiatica, Vitamins, Glycolic Acid and Their Mixtures Preparations in Stimulating Collagen and Fibronectin Synthesis in Cultured Human Skin Fibroblast." *Pak J Pharm Sci* 27, no. 2 (March 2014): 2337. https://www.ncbi.nlm.nih.gov/pubmed/24577907.

CHROMIUM

Hehenberger, K., et al. "Inhibited Proliferation of Fibroblasts Derived from Chronic Diabetic Wounds and Normal Dermal Fibroblasts Treated with High Glucose Is Associated with Increased Formation of l-lactate." *Wound Repair Regen* 6 (1998): 135–41.

Spravchikov, N., et al. "Glucose Effects on Skin Keratinocytes: Implications for Diabetes Skin Complications." *Diabetes* 50 (2001) 1627–35.

COENZYME Q10

Blatt, T. and G. P. Litarru. "Biochemical Rationale and Experimental Data on the Anti-aging Properties of CoQ10 at Skin Level." *Biofactors* 37, no. 5 (September–October 2011): 381–85.

Zhang, M., et al. "Coenzyme Q10 Enhances Dermal Elastin Expression, Inhibits IL-1a Production and Melanin Synthesis in Vivo." *Int J Cosmet Sci* 34, no. 3 (June 2012): 273–79.

COFFEE POLYPHENOLS

Fukagawa S., et al. "Coffee Polyphenols Extracted from Green Coffee Beans Improve Skin Properties and Microcirculatory Function." *Biosci Biotechnol Biochem* 81, no. 9 (September 2017): 1814–22. doi: 10.1080/09168451. 2017.1345614. Epub July 4, 2017. https://www.ncbi.nlm.nih.gov/pubmed/28675091.

CURCUMIN

https://www.ncbi.nlm.nih.gov/pubmed/23231506.

Agrawal, R., and I. P. Kaur. "Inhibitory Effect of Encapsulated Curcumin on Ultraviolet-Induced Photoaging in Mice." *Rejuvenation Res* 13, no. 4 (August 2010): 397–410. doi: 10.1089/rej.2009.0906. https://www.ncbi.nlm.nih.gov/pubmed/20938987.

Li, X, et al. "EGF and Curcumin Co-encapsulated Nanoparticle/Hydrogel System as Potent Skin Regeneration Agent." *Int. J Nanomedicine* 11 (August 17, 2016): 3993–4009. doi: 10.2147/IJN.S104350. eCollection 2016. https://www.ncbi.nlm.nih.gov/pubmed/20618464.

Mukherjee, P. K., et al. "Bioactive Compounds From Natural Resources Against Skin Aging." *Phytomedicine* 19, no. 1 (December 15, 2011): 64–73. doi: 10.1016/j.phymed.2011.10.003. Epub November 23, 2011.

Panchatcharam, M., et al. "Curcumin Improves Wound Healing by Modulating Collagen and Decreasing Reactive Oxygen Species." *Mol Cell Biochem* 290 (2006): 87–96. https://www.ncbi.nlm.nih.gov/pubmed/16770527.

GENISTEIN

Polito, F., et al. "Genistein Aglycone, a Soy-Derived Isoflavone, Improves Skin Changes in Ovariectomy in Rats." *Br J Pharmacol* 165, no. 4 (February 2012): 994–1005. doi: 10.1111/j.1476-5381.2011.01619.x.

Silva, L. A., et al. "Collagen Concentration on the Facial Skin of Post-menopausal women After Topical Treatment of Estradiol and Genistein: A Randomized Double-Blind Controlled Trial." *Gynecol Endocrinol*, 33, no. 11 (November 2017): 845–48. doi: 10.1080/09513590.2017.1320708. Epub May 16, 2017.

Waqas, M. K., et al. "Dermatological and Cosmeceutical Benefits of Glycine Max (Soybean) and Its Active Components." *Acta Pol Pharm* 72, no. 1 (January–February 2015): 3–11.

GLUCOSAMINE

Gueniche, A. and I. Castiel-Higounenc. "Efficacy of Glucosamine Sulphate in Skin Ageing: Results from an Ex-Vivo Anti-ageing Model in a Clinical Trial." *Skin Pharmacol Physiol* 30, no. 1 (2017): 36–41.

Hwang, Y. P., et al. "N-Acetyl-Glucosamine Suppress Collagenase Activation in Ultraviolet B-Irradiated Human Dermal Fibroblasts: Involvement of Calcium Ions and Mitogen-Activated Protein Kinases." *J Dermatol Sci* 63, no. 2 (August 2011): 93–103.

HYALURONIC ACID

Papakonstantinou, E., M. Roth, and G. Karakiulakis. "Hyaluronic Acid: A Key Molecule in Skin Aging." *Dermatoendocrinol* 4, no. 3 (July 1, 2012): 253–58. https://www.ncbi.nlm.nih.gov/pmc/articles/PMC3583886/.

IRON

Wright, Josephine, Toby Richards, and Surjit Srai. "The Role of Iron in the Skin and Cutaneous Wound Healing." *Front Pharmacol* 5 (2014): 156. https://www.ncbi.nlm.nih.gov/pmc/articles/PMC4091310/.

LYCOPENE

Basavarai, K. H., et al. "Diet in Dermatology: Present Perspectives." *Indian J Dermatol* 55, no. 3 (July–September 2010): 205–21. https://www.ncbi.nlm.nih.gov/pmc/articles/PMC2965901/.

Chiang, H. S., et al. "Lycopene Inhibits PDGF-BB-Induced Signaling and Migration in Human Dermal Fibroblasts Through Interaction with PDGF-BB." *Life Sci* 81, no. 21–22 (November 10, 2007): 1509–17. Epub October 2, 2007.

Costa, A., et al. "Clinical, Biometric and Ultrasound Assessment of the Effects of Daily Use of a Nutraceutical Composed of Lycopene, Acerola Extract, Grape Seed Extract and Biomarine Complex in Photoaged Human Skin." *An Bras Dermatol* 87, no. 1 (January–February 2012): 52–81. https://www.ncbi.nlm.nih.gov/pubmed/?term=Costa+A1%2C+Lindmark+L%2C+Arruda+LH%2C.

159

MAGNESIUM

Grober, Uwe, et al. "Myth or Reality—Transdermal Magnesium." *Nutrients* 9, no. 8 (August 2017): 813. https://www.ncbi.nlm.nih.gov/pmc/articles/PMC5579607/.

OMEGA-3 FATTY ACIDS

Basavarai, K. H., et al. "Diet in Dermatology: Present Perspectives." *Indian J Dermatol* 55, no. 3 (July–September 2010): 205–21. https://www.ncbi.nlm.nih.gov/pmc/articles/PMC2965901/.

Kim, H. H., et al. "Photoprotective and Anti-Skin-Aging Effects of Eicosapentaenoic Acid in Human Skin in Vivo." *J Lipid Res May* 47, no. 5 (2006): 921–30. Epub February 7, 2006.

Oikawa, D., et al. "Dietary CLA and DHA Modify Skin Properties in Mice." *Lipids* 38, no. 6 (June 2003): 609–14. https://www.ncbi.nlm.nih.gov/pubmed/?term=Dietary+CLA+and+DHA+modify+skin+properties+in+mice.

PROBIOTICS

Fabbrocini, G., et al. "Supplementation with Lactobacillus rhamnosus SP1 Normalises Skin Expression of Genes Implicated in Insulin Signalling and Improves Adult Acne." *Benef Microbes* 7, no. 5 (November 30, 2016): 625–30. https://www.ncbi.nlm.nih.gov/pubmed/?term=probiotics+skin+collagen.

Kim H., et al. "Effects of Oral Intake of Kimchi-Derived Lactobacillus plantarum K8 Lysates on Skin Moisturizing." *J Microbiol Biotechnol* 25, no. 1 (January 2015): 74–80.

Kim H. M., et al. "Oral Administration of Lactobacillus plantarum HY7714 Protects Hairless Mouse Against Ultraviolet B-Induced Photoaging." *J Microbiol Biotechnol* 24, no. 11 (November 28, 2014): 1583–91. https://www.ncbi.nlm.nih.gov/pubmed/?term=probiotics+skin+collagen.

Jeong J. H., C. Y. Lee, and D. K. Chung. "Probiotic Lactic Acid Bacteria and Skin Health." *Crit Rev Food Sci Nut* 56, no. 14 (October 25, 2016): 2331–37. doi: 10.1080/10408398.2013.834874. https://www.ncbi.nlm.nih.gov/pubmed/27596801.

Muizzuddin, N, W. Maher, M. Sullivan, S. Schnittger, and T. Mammone. "Physiological Effect of a Probiotic on Skin." *J Cosmet Sci* 63, no. 6 (November–December 2012): 385–95.

POMEGRANATE

Aggarwal, B. B. and S Shishodia. "Suppression of the Nuclear Factor-Kappa B Activation Pathway by Spice Derived Phytochemicals: Reasoning for Seasoning." *Ann NY Acad Sci* 1030 (2004): 434–41. https://www.ncbi.nlm.nih.gov/pubmed/15659827.

Park, H. M., et al. "Extract of Punica granatum Inhibits Skin Photoaging Induced by UVB Irradiation." *Int J Dermatol* 49, no. 3 (March 2010): 276–82. doi: 10.1111/j.1365-4632.2009.04269.x.

RESVERATROL

Farris, P., et al. "Evaluation of Efficacy and Tolerance of a Nighttime Topical Antioxidant Containing Resveratrol, Baicalin, and Vitamin E for Treatment of Mild to Moderate Photodamaged Skin." *J Drugs Dermatol* 13, no. 12 (December 2014): 1467–72.

Ikeda, K., et al. "Resveratrol Inhibits Fibrogenesis and Induces Apoptosis in Keloid Fibroblasts." *Wound Repair Regen* 21, no. 4 (July–August 2013): 616–23. doi: 10.1111/wrr.12062.

Mamalis, A. and J. Jagdeo. "The Combination of Resveratrol and High-Fluence Light-Emitting Diode-Red Light Produces Synergistic Photobotanical Inhibition of Fibroblast Proliferation and Collagen Synthesis: A Novel Treatment for Skin Fibrosis." *Dermatol Surg* 43, no. 1 (January 2017): 81–86. doi: 10.1097/DSS.0000000000000921.

Wittenauer, J., et al. "Inhibitory Effects of Polyphenols from Grape Pomace Extract on Collagenase and Elastase Activity." *Fitoterpia* 101 (March 2015): 179–87. doi: 10.1016/j.fitote.2015.01.005. Epub January 15, 2015.

Zeng, G., et al. "Resveratrol-Mediated Reduction of Collagen by Inhibiting Proliferation and Producing Apoptosis in Human Hypertrophic Scar Fibroblasts." *Biosci Biotechnol Biochem* 77, no. 12 (2013): 2389–96. Epub December 7, 2013.

Zhao, P., et al. "Anti-aging Pharmacology in Cutaneous Wound Healing: Effects of Metformin, Resveratrol, and Rapamycin by Local Application." *Aging Cell* 16, no. 5 (October 2017): 1083–93. doi: 10.1111/acel.12635. Epub July 5, 2017.

SELENIUM

Basavarai, K. H., et al. "Diet in Dermatology: Present Perspectives." *Indian J Dermatol* 55, no. 3 (July–September 2010): 205–21. https://www.ncbi.nlm.nih.gov/pmc/articles/PMC2965901/.

SULFUR

"Sulfur." University of Maryland Medical Center. Accessed March 3, 2018. https://www.umm.edu/health/medical/altmed/supplement/sulfur.

VITAMIN A

Basavarai, K. H., et al. "Diet in Dermatology: Present Perspectives." *Indian J Dermatol* 55, no. 3 (July–September 2010): 205–21. https://www.ncbi.nlm.nih.gov/pmc/articles/PMC2965901/.

"Vitamin A." The World's Healthiest Foods. Accessed February 25, 2018. http://www.whfoods.com/genpage.php?tname=nutrient&dbid=106.

VITAMIN B$_3$

Bissett, D. L., J. E. Oblong, and C. A. Berge. "Niacinamide: A B Vitamin That Improves Aging Facial Skin Appearance." *Dermatol Surg* 31, no. 7, pt. 2 (July 2005): 860–65.

Chen, A. C., et al. "A Phase 3 Randomized Trial of Nicotinamide for Skin-Cancer Chemoprevention." *N Engl J Med* 373, no. 17 (October 22, 2015): 1618–28. https://www.ncbi.nlm.nih.gov/pubmed/26488693.

Esfahani, S., et al. "Topical Nicotinamide Improves Tissue Regeneration in Excisional Full-Thickness Skin Wounds: A Stereological and Pathological Study." *Trauma Mon* 20, no. 4 (November 2015): e18193. https://www.ncbi.nlm.nih.gov/pmc/articles/PMC4727459/.

Ganceviciene, R. et al. "Skin Anti-aging Strategies." *Dermatoendocrinol* 4, no. 3 (July 1, 2012): 308–19. https://www.ncbi.nlm.nih.gov/pmc/articles/PMC3583892/.

VITAMIN B$_7$ (BIOTIN)

"Biotin." Oregon State University. Linus Pauling Institute. Micronutrient Information Center. Accessed March 4, 2018. http://lpi.oregonstate.edu/mic/vitamins/biotin.

VITAMIN B$_9$ (FOLIC ACID, OR FOLATE)

Williams, J.D., et al. "Folate in Skin Cancer Prevention." *Subcell Biochem* 56 (2012): 181–97. https://www.ncbi.nlm.nih.gov/pmc/articles/PMC3795437/.

VITAMIN B$_{12}$

Basavarai, K. H., et al. "Diet in Dermatology: Present Perspectives. *Indian J Dermatol* 55, no. 3 (July–September 2010): 205–21." https://www.ncbi.nlm.nih.gov/pmc/articles/PMC2965901/.

VITAMIN C

Basavarai, K. H., et al. "Diet in Dermatology: Present Perspectives." *Indian J Dermatol* 55, no. 3, (July–September 2010): 205–21. https://www.ncbi.nlm.nih.gov/pmc/articles/PMC2965901/.

Campos, P. M., G. M. Goncalves, and L. R. Gaspar. "In Vitro Antioxidant Activity and In Vivo Efficacy of Topical Formulations Containing Vitamin C and Its Derivatives Studied by Non-invasive Methods." *Skin Res Technol* 14 (2008): 376–80.

Peterkofsky, B. "Ascorbate Requirement for Hydroxylation and Secretion of Procollagen: Relationship to Inhibition of Collagen Synthesis in Scurvy." *Am J Clin Nutr* 54 (1991): 1135s–1140s.

Ross, R. and E. P. Benditt. "Wound Healing and Collagen Formation. II. Fine Structure in Experimental Scurvy." *Cell Biol* 12 (1962): 533–51.

VITAMIN E

Basavarai, K. H., et al. "Diet in Dermatology: Present Perspectives." *Indian J Dermatol* 55, no. 3) July–September 2010): 205–21. https://www.ncbi.nlm.nih.gov/pmc/articles/PMC2965901/.

Burke, K. E., et al. "Effects of Topical and Oral Vitamin E on Pigmentation and Skin Cancer Induced by Ultraviolet Irradiation in Skh:2 Hairless Mice." *Nutr Cancer* 38 (2000): 87–97.

Ganceviciene, R. et al. "Skin Anti-aging Strategies." *Dermatoendocrinol* 4, no. 3 (July 1, 2012): 308–19. https://www.ncbi.nlm.nih.gov/pmc/articles/PMC3583892/.

Lin, J. Y., et al. "UV Photoprotection by Combination Topical Antioxidants Vitamin C and Vitamin E." *J Am Acad Dermatol* 48 (2003): 866–74.

Meydani, S. N., et al. "Vitamin E Supplementation Enhances Cell Mediated Immunity in Healthy Elderly Subjects." *Am J Clin Nutr* 52 (1990): 557–63.

Steenvoorden, D. P. and Beijersbergen van Henegouwen. "Protection Against UV-Induced Systemic Immunosuppression in Mice by a Single Topical Application of the Antioxidant Vitamins C and E." *Radiat Biol* 75 (1999): 747–55.

Thiele, J. J., M. G. Traber, L. and Packer. "Depletion of Human Stratum Corneum Vitamin E: An Early and Sensitive In Vivo Marker of UV Induced Photo-oxidation." *J Invest Dermatol* 110 (1998): 756–61.

Tyrrell, R. M. and S. M. Keyse. "New Trends in Photobiology. The Interaction of UVA Radiation with Cultured Cells." *J Photochem Photobiol B* 4 (1990): 349–61.

Wu, S., et al. "IL-8 Production and AP-1 Transactivation Induced by UVA in Human Keratinocytes: Roles of D-Alpha-Tocopherol." *Mol Immunol* 45 (2008): 2288–96.

ZINC

Basavarai, K. H., et al. "Diet in Dermatology: Present Perspectives." *Indian J Dermatol* 55, no. 3 (July–September 2010): 205–21. https://www.ncbi.nlm.nih.gov/pmc/articles/PMC2965901/.

Mitchnick, M. A., et al. "Microfine Zinc Oxide (Z-cote) as a Photostable UVA/UVB Sunblock Agent." *J Am Acad Dermatol* 40 (1999): 85–90.

REFERENCES FOR FEATURED INGREDIENTS

Ali, B. H., et al. "The Effect of Activated Charcoal on Adenine-Induced Chronic Renal Failure in Rats." *Food and Chemical Toxicology* 65 (2014): 321–28.

Altman, R. D., and K. C. Marcussen. "Effects of a Ginger Extract on Knee Pain in Patients with Osteoarthritis." *Arthritis and Rheumatism* 44, no. 11 (2001): 2531–38.

Amagase, H., and D. M. Nance. "A Randomized, Double-Blind, Placebo-Controlled, Clinical Study of the General Effects of a Standardized Lycium Barbarum (Goji) Juice, Gochi (Tm)." *Journal of Alternative and Complementary Medicine* 14, no. 4 (2008): 403–12.

Asha'ari, Z. A., et al. "Ingestion of Honey Improves the Symptoms of Allergic Rhinitis: Evidence from a Randomized Placebo-Controlled Trial in the East Coast of Peninsular Malaysia." *Annals of Saudi Medicine* 33, no. 5 (2013): 469–75.

Basu, A., M. Rhone, and T. J. Lyons. "Berries: Emerging Impact on Cardiovascular Health." *Nutrition Reviews* 68, no. 3 (2010): 168–77.

Binic, I., et al. "Skin Ageing: Natural Weapons and Strategies." *Evidence-Based Complementary and Alternative Medicine* (2013).

Black, C. D., et al. "Ginger (Zingiber Officinale) Reduces Muscle Pain Caused by Eccentric Exercise." *Journal of Pain* 11, no. 9 (2010): 894–903.

Boots, A. W., G. R. M. M. Haenen, and A. Bast. "Health Effects of Quercetin: From Antioxidant to Nutraceutical." *European Journal of Pharmacology* 585, no. 2–3 (2008): 325–37.

Boskabady, M. H., et al. "Pharmacological Effects of Rosa Damascena." *Iranian Journal of Basic Medical Sciences* 14, no. 4 (2011): 295–307.

Carey, A. N., et al. "Dietary Supplementation with the Polyphenol-Rich Acai Pulps (Euterpe Oleracea Mart. and Euterpe Precatoria Mart.) Improves Cognition in Aged Rats and Attenuates Inflammatory Signaling in Bv-2 Microglial Cells." *Nutritional Neuroscience* 20, no. 4 (2017): 238–45.

Chainani-Wu, N. "Safety and Anti-Inflammatory Activity of Curcumin: A Component of Tumeric (Curcuma Longa)." *Journal of Alternative and Complementary Medicine* 9, no. 1 (2003): 161–68.

Clifton, P. M., J. B. Keogh, and M. Noakes. "Long-Term Effects of a High-Protein Weight-Loss Diet." *American Journal of Clinical Nutrition* 87, no. 1 (2008): 23–29.

Corti, R., et al. "Cocoa and Cardiovascular Health." *Circulation* 119, no. 10 (2009): 1433–41.

Delcourt, C., et al. "Plasma Lutein and Zeaxanthin and Other Carotenoids as Modifiable Risk Factors for Age-Related Maculopathy and Cataract: The Pola Study." *Investigative Ophthalmology & Visual Science* 47, no. 6 (2006): 2329–35.

Deng, H. B., et al. "Inhibiting Effects of Achyranthes Bidentata Polysaccharide and Lycium Barbarum Polysaccharide on Nonenzyme Glycation in D-Galactose Induced Mouse Aging Model." *Biomedical and Environmental Sciences* 16, no. 3 (2003): 267–75.

Ernst, E., and M. H. Pittler. "Efficacy of Ginger for Nausea and Vomiting: A Systematic Review of Randomized Clinical Trials." *British Journal of Anaesthesia* 84, no. 3 (2000): 367–71.

Fang, C., et al. "Mango Polyphenols (Mangifera Indica L.) and Their Microbial Metabolites Suppress Adipogenesis and Fat Accumulation by Mediating Ampk Signaling Pathways in 3t3l-1 Adipocytes." *Faseb Journal* 30 (2016).

Feio, C. M., et al. "Euterpe Oleracea (Acai) Modifies Sterol Metabolism and Attenuates Experimentally-Induced Atherosclerosis." *Circulation* 125, no. 19 (2012): E924-E24.

Forastiere, F., et al. "Consumption of Fresh Fruit Rich in Vitamin C and Wheezing Symptoms in Children." *Thorax* 55, no. 4 (2000): 283–88.

French, D. L., J. M. Muir, and C. E. Webber. "The Ovariectomized, Mature Rat Model of Postmenopausal Osteoporosis: An Assessment of the Bone Sparing Effects of Curcumin." *Phytomedicine* 15, no. 12 (2008): 1069–78.

Fukuchi, Y., et al. "Lemon Polyphenols Suppress Diet-Induced Obesity by Up-Regulation of Mrna Levels of the Enzymes Involved in Beta-Oxidation in Mouse White Adipose Tissue." *Journal of Clinical Biochemistry and Nutrition* 43, no. 3 (2008): 201–9.

Ganji, S. H., V. S. Kamanna, and M. L. Kashyap. "Niacin and Cholesterol: Role in Cardiovascular Disease (Review)." *Journal of Nutritional Biochemistry* 14, no. 6 (2003): 298–305.

Gorinstein, S., et al. "Comparative Content of Total Polyphenols and Dietary Fiber in Tropical Fruits and Persimmon." *Journal of Nutritional Biochemistry* 10, no. 6 (1999): 367–71.

Grogan, S. P., and E. A. Egitto. "Honey for Acute Cough in Children." *American Family Physician* 94, no. 1 (2016): 20–21.

Hanson, M. G., P. Zahradka, and C. G. Taylor. "Lentil-Based Diets Attenuate Hypertension and Large-Artery Remodelling in Spontaneously Hypertensive Rats." *British Journal of Nutrition* 111, no. 4 (2014): 690–98.

Homnava, A., et al. "Provitamin-a (Alpha-Carotene, Beta-Carotene and Beta-Cryptoxanthin) and Ascorbic-Acid Content of Japanese and American Persimmons." *Journal of Food Quality* 13, no. 2 (1990): 85–95.

Jalal, F., et al. "Serum Retinol Concentrations in Children Are Affected by Food Sources of Beta-Carotene, Fat Intake, and Anthelmintic Drug Treatment." *American Journal of Clinical Nutrition* 68, no. 3 (1998): 623–29.

Joshi, R., et al. "Free Radical Scavenging Behavior of Folic Acid: Evidence for Possible Antioxidant Activity." *Free Radical Biology and Medicine* 30, no. 12 (2001): 1390–99.

Josling, P. "Preventing the Common Cold with a Garlic Supplement: A Double-Blind, Placebo-Controlled Survey." *Advances in Therapy* 18, no. 4 (2001): 189_93.

Kahlon, T. S., M. C. M. Chiu, and M. H. Chapman. "Steam Cooking Significantly Improves in Vitro Bile Acid Binding of Collard Greens, Kale, Mustard Greens, Broccoli, Green Bell Pepper, and Cabbage." *Nutrition Research* 28, no. 6 (2008): 351–57.

Kaur, L., et al. "Actinidin Enhances Gastric Protein Digestion as Assessed Using an in Vitro Gastric Digestion Model." *Journal of Agricultural and Food Chemistry* 58, no. 8 (2010): 5068–73.

Khan, A., et al. "Cinnamon Improves Glucose and Lipids of People with Type 2 Diabetes." *Diabetes Care* 26, no. 12 (2003): 3215–18.

Kondo, T., et al. "Vinegar Intake Reduces Body Weight, Body Fat Mass, and Serum Triglyceride Levels in Obese Japanese Subjects." *Bioscience Biotechnology and Biochemistry* 73, no. 8 (2009): 1837–43.

Krasopoulos, J. C., V. A. Debari, and M. A. Needle. "The Adsorption of Bile-Salts on Activated Carbon." *Lipids* 15, no. 5 (1980): 365–70.

Lee, J. C., et al. "Marine Algal Natural Products with Anti-Oxidative, Anti-Inflammatory, and Anti-cancer Properties." *Cancer Cell International* 13 (2013).

Liu, X., et al. "Cordyceps Sinensis Protects Against Liver and Heart Injuries in a Rat Model of Chronic Kidney Disease: A Metabolomic Analysis." *Acta Pharmacologica Sinica* 35, no. 5 (2014): 697–706.

Mazokopakis, E. E., et al. "The Hypolipidaemic Effects of Spirulina (Arthrospira Platensis) Supplementation in a Cretan Population: A Prospective Study." *Journal of the Science of Food and Agriculture* 94, no. 3 (2014): 432–37.

Miyazaki, Y., et al. "Effects on Immune Response of Antidiabetic Ingredients from White-Skinned Sweet Potato (Ipomoea Batatas L.)." *Nutrition* 21, no. 3 (2005): 358–62.

Morand, C., et al. "Hesperidin Contributes to the Vascular Protective Effects of Orange Juice: A Randomized Crossover Study in Healthy Volunteers." *American Journal of Clinical Nutrition* 93, no. 1 (2011): 73–80.

Moser, B., et al. "Impact of Spinach Consumption on DNA Stability in Peripheral Lymphocytes and on Biochemical Blood Parameters: Results of a Human Intervention Trial." *European Journal of Nutrition* 50, no. 7 (2011): 587–94.

Naz, A., et al. "Watermelon Lycopene and Allied Health Claims." *Excli Journal* 13 (2014): 650–66.

Pengelly, A., et al. "Short-Term Study on the Effects of Rosemary on Cognitive Function in an Elderly Population." *Journal of Medicinal Food* 15, no. 1 (2012): 10–17.

Rao, P. V., and S. H. Gan. "Cinnamon: A Multifaceted Medicinal Plant." *Evidence-Based Complementary and Alternative Medicine* (2014).

Resnick, E. S., B. P. Bielory, and L. Bielory. "Complementary Therapy in Allergic Rhinitis." *Current Allergy and Asthma Reports* 8, no. 2 (2008): 118–25.

Riso, P., et al. "Effect of a Wild Blueberry (Vaccinium Angustifolium) Drink Intervention on Markers of Oxidative Stress, Inflammation and Endothelial Function in Humans with Cardiovascular Risk Factors." *European Journal of Nutrition* 52, no. 3 (2013): 949–61.

Seth, A., et al. "Potassium Intake and Risk of Stroke in Women with Hypertension and Nonhypertension in the Women's Health Initiative." *Stroke* 45, no. 10 (2014): 2874–80.

Stoner, G. D., et al. "Carcinogen-Altered Genes in Rat Esophagus Positively Modulated to Normal Levels of Expression by Both Black Raspberries and Phenylethyl Isothiocyanate." *Cancer Research* 68, no. 15 (2008): 6460–67.

Svendsen, M., et al. "The Effect of Kiwifruit Consumption on Blood Pressure in Subjects with Moderately Elevated Blood Pressure: A Randomized, Controlled Study." *Blood Pressure* 24, no. 1 (2015): 48–54.

Tai, J., et al. "Antiproliferation Effect of Rosemary (Rosmarinus Officinalis) on Human Ovarian Cancer Cells in Vitro." *Phytomedicine* 19, no. 5 (2012): 436–43.

Taing, M. W., et al. "Mango Fruit Peel and Flesh Extracts Affect Adipogenesis in 3t3-L1 Cells." *Food & Function* 3, no. 8 (2012): 828–36.

Taub, P. R., et al. "Alterations in Skeletal Muscle Indicators of Mitochondrial Structure and Biogenesis in Patients with Type 2 Diabetes and Heart Failure: Effects of Epicatechin Rich Cocoa." *Cts-Clinical and Translational Science* 5, no. 1 (2012): 43–47.

Thring, T. S. A., P. Hili, and D. P. Naughton. "Antioxidant and Potential Anti-Inflammatory Activity of Extracts and Formulations of White Tea, Rose, and Witch Hazel on Primary Human Dermal Fibroblast Cells." *Journal of Inflammation-London* 8 (2011).

Torronen, R., et al. "Berries Modify the Postprandial Plasma Glucose Response to Sucrose in Healthy Subjects." *British Journal of Nutrition* 103, no. 8 (2010): 1094–97.

Udani, J. K., et al. "Effects of Acai (Euterpe Oleracea Mart.) Berry Preparation on Metabolic Parameters in a Healthy Overweight Population: A Pilot Study." *Nutrition Journal* 10 (2011).

Vieira, A. J., F. P. Beserra, M. C. Souza, B. M. Totti, and A. L. Rozza. "Limonene: Aroma of Innovation in Health and Disease." *Chemico-Biological Interactions* 283 (2018).

Wabner, C. L., and C. Y. C. Pak. "Effect of Orange Juice Consumption on Urinary Stone Risk-Factors." *Journal of Urology* 149, no. 6 (1993): 1405–8.

Watson, R. R., et al. "Oral Administration of the Purple Passion Fruit Peel Extract Reduces Wheeze and Cough and Improves Shortness of Breath in Adults with Asthma." *Nutrition Research* 28, no. 3 (2008): 166–71.

Williams, F. M. K., et al. "Dietary Garlic and Hip Osteoarthritis: Evidence of a Protective Effect and Putative Mechanism of Action." *Bmc Musculoskeletal Disorders* 11 (2010).

Xia, H. C., et al. "Purification and Characterization of Moschatin, a Novel Type I Ribosomeinactivating Protein from the Mature Seeds of Pumpkin (Cucurbita Moschata), and Preparation of Its Immunotoxin against Human Melanoma Cells." *Cell Research* 13, no. 5 (2003): 369–74.

STUDIES

- In 2015, Jérome Asserin and his colleagues published the results of two placebo-controlled clinical trials to assess daily oral supplementation with collagen peptides. The studies found that oral collagen peptide significantly increased skin hydration after eight weeks of intake, as well as the collagen density in the dermis, while collagen fragmentation decreased (results occurred after four weeks). All these effects continued after 12 weeks.

- A 2008 study in Tokyo of 33 women aged forty to sixty who took 10 g of hydrolyzed collagen daily for two months showed a 91 percent increase in skin hydration and resilience.

- A Dermscan study in Lyon, France, in 2008 showed similar findings in a group of participants aged thirty-five to fifty-five: an increase in skin smoothness and hydration. After 12 weeks of 10 g hydrolyzed collagen daily, the subjects had 41 percent less furrowing and fewer wrinkles, and were more resilient and more hydrated.

- As measured by the C&Z Cutometer, hydrolyzed collagen increases the diameter of collagen fibrils in the dermis via fibroblast stimulation. This in turn increases cohesion of the dermal collagen fibers themselves, which translates to increased thickness, suppleness, and resilience of skin.

- Double-blind, placebo-controlled studies investigating the antiaging properties of collagen have found that 2.5 to 5 grams of collagen hydrolysate used among women aged thirty-five to fifty-five once daily for eight weeks significantly improved skin elasticity, skin moisture, transepidermal water loss (dryness), and skin roughness.

- A study published in the *Journal of Investigative Dermatology* noted "essential relationships between extracellular matrix (ECM) and hair follicle regeneration, suggesting that collagen could be a potential therapeutic target for hair loss and other skin-related diseases."

169

INDEX

171

175

ABOUT THE AUTHOR

Sally Olivia Kim discovered the power of ingestible skincare after experiencing painful burns up and down both of her arms. When topical creams and ointments didn't work, she decided to try drinking collagen to see if it could help speed her recovery. Soon, she was seeing results, and not just in her arms: her hair seemed thicker and stronger and she no longer was struggling with dry skin and dark circles under her eyes.

Excited about her own results, Sally started recommending ingestible collagen to friends and family; yet due to the taste of collagen when taken by itself, no one wanted to take it as consistently as Sally had.

This sparked Sally's passion in bringing the benefits of collagen to everyone she loved, and she started formulating recipes using collagen as a base of many of her drinks.

After months and months of testing multiple types of collagen and tasting it with various superfoods in the kitchen, Sally was finally able to get everyone around her to be just as hooked on collagen as she is—and that's when Crushed Tonic was born.